THE ESSENTIAL
Aromatherapy
BOOK

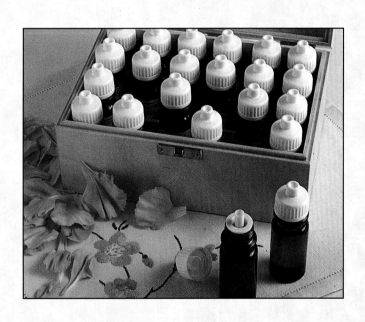

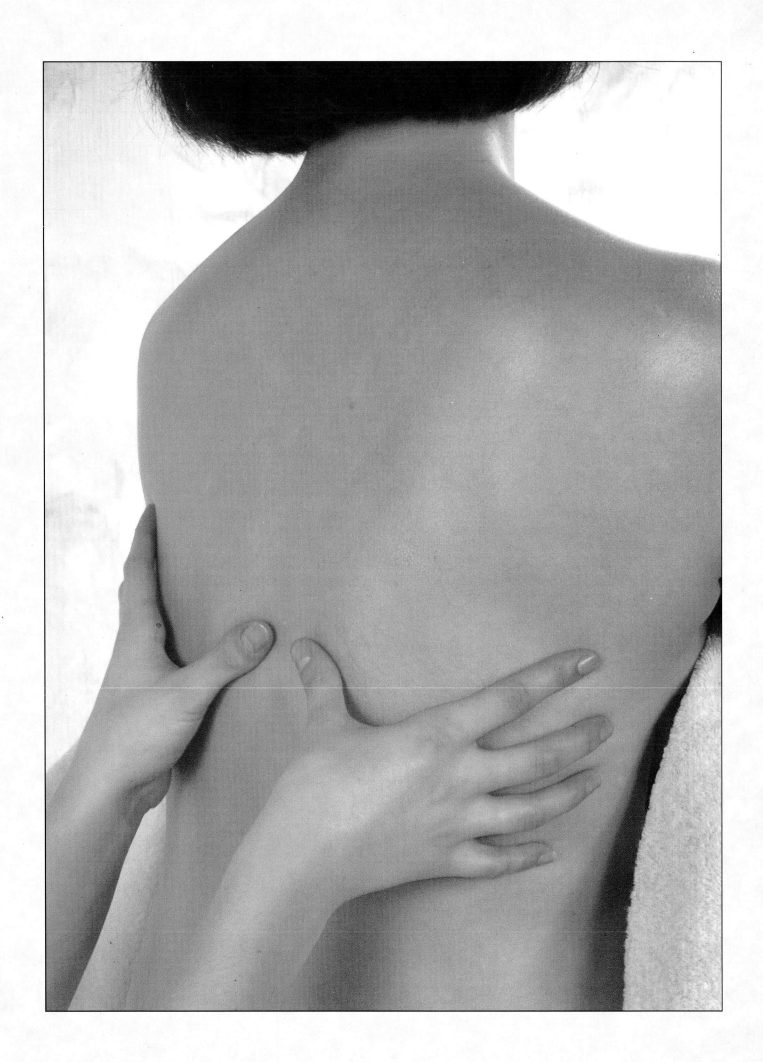

THE ESSENTIAL
Aromatherapy
BOOK

CAROLE McGILVERY & JIMI REED

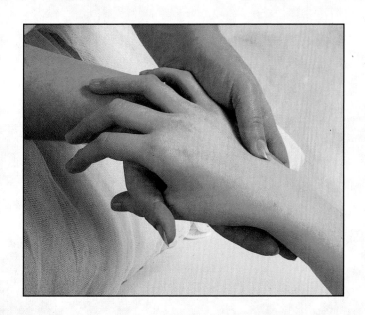

Photography by
SUE ATKINSON

HERMES
HOUSE

This edition published by Hermes House
an imprint of
Anness Publishing Limited
Hermes House
88-89 Blackfriars Road
London SE1 8HA

Published in the USA by Hermes House
Anness Publishing Inc., 27 West 20th Street, New York, NY 10011;
(800) 354-9657

ISBN 1 84038 406 9

A CIP catalogue record for this book is available from the British Library

Publisher: Joanna Lorenz
Photography: Sue Atkinson
Photographic Assistant: Kirsty Wilson
Designer: Kit Johnson
Artwork: Raymond Turvey
Production Controller: Joanna Simmons

Printed in Singapore by Star Standard Industries Pte. Ltd.

Also published as part of a larger compendium,
The Encyclopedia of Aromatherapy, Massage and Yoga

© Anness Publishing Limited 1995, 1998
Updated © 1999
1 3 5 7 9 10 8 6 4 2

PICTURE CREDITS

The Bridgeman Art Library: p. 8, top and below
Picturepoint Ltd: pp. 9 and 10-11
French Picture Library: p. 11, inset below
Ancient Art and Architecture Collection: p. 11, inset top

PUBLISHER'S NOTE

The reader should not regard the recommendations, ideas and techniques
expressed and described in this book as substitutes for the advice of a
qualified medical practitioner. Any use to which the recommendations,
ideas and techniques are put is at the reader's sole discretion and risk.

CONTENTS

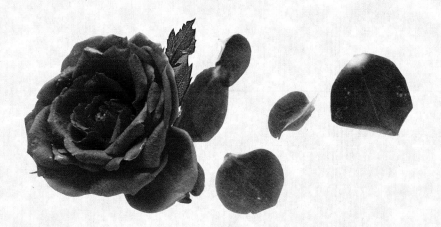

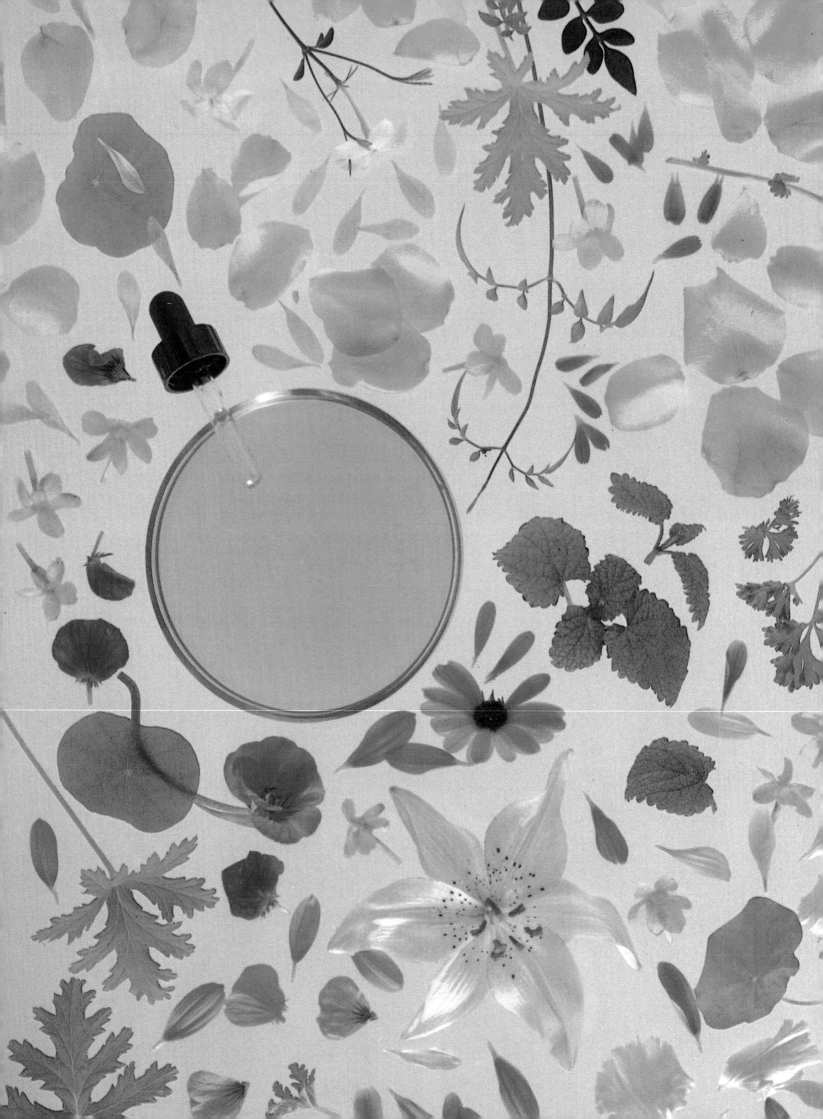

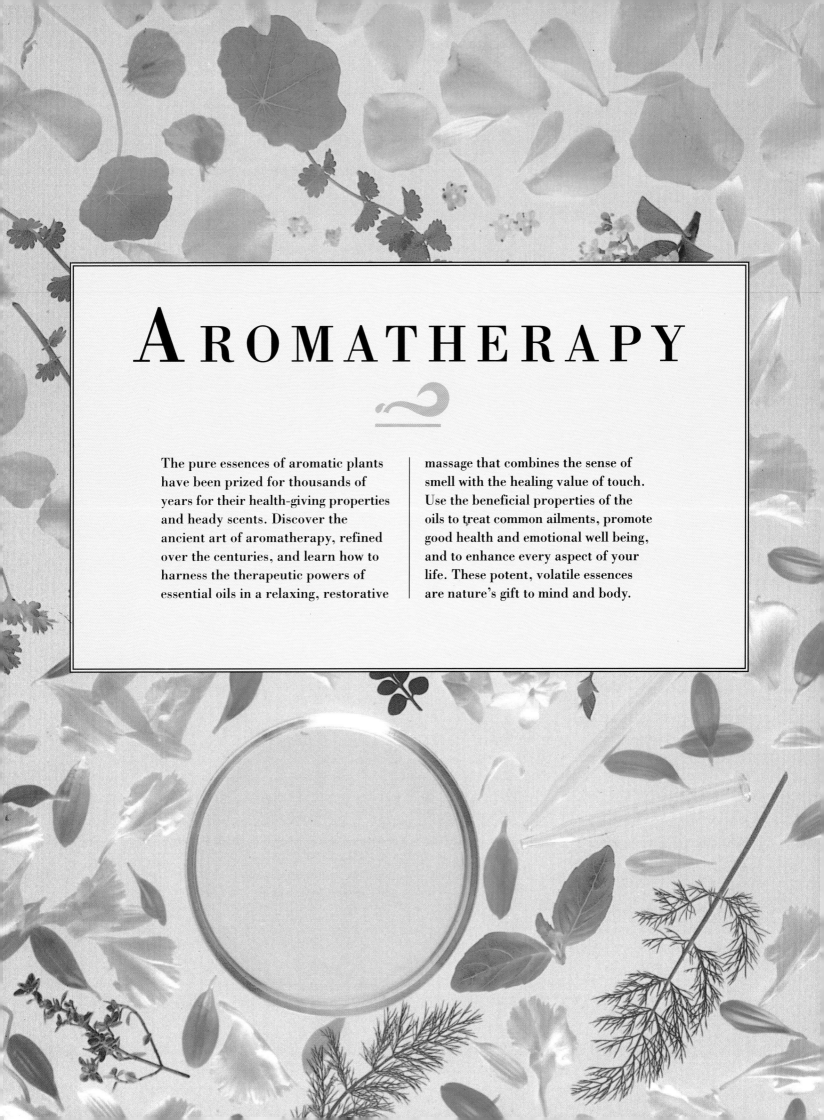

AROMATHERAPY

The pure essences of aromatic plants have been prized for thousands of years for their health-giving properties and heady scents. Discover the ancient art of aromatherapy, refined over the centuries, and learn how to harness the therapeutic powers of essential oils in a relaxing, restorative massage that combines the sense of smell with the healing value of touch. Use the beneficial properties of the oils to treat common ailments, promote good health and emotional well being, and to enhance every aspect of your life. These potent, volatile essences are nature's gift to mind and body.

AN ANCIENT ART

The value of natural plant oils has been recognized for more than 6000 years, for their healing, cleansing, preservative and mood-enhancing properties, as well as for the sheer pleasure of their fragrances. Today, these properties are being rediscovered as we look to the wisdom of past eras and civilizations to restore the balance that has been lost in modern-day life. Stress, pollution, unhealthy diet, hectic but sedentary lifestyles – all these factors have adverse effects on our bodies and spirits. The art of aromatherapy harnesses the potent pure essences of aromatic plants, flowers and resins, to work on the most powerful of senses – smell and touch – to restore the harmony of body and mind.

SECRETS OF THE OILS DISCOVERED

The origins of aromatherapy can be traced through the religious, medical and social practices of all the major civilizations. It is likely that the Chinese were the first to discover the remarkable medicinal powers of plants around 4500 BC. However, it is the Egyptians who must take the credit for recognizing and fully exploiting the physical and spiritual properties of aromatic essences. From hieroglyphs and paintings we know that aromatic preparations were used as offerings to the gods. Furthermore the natural antiseptic and antibacterial properties of essential oils and resins, particularly cedarwood and frankincense, made them ideal for the purpose of preserving corpses in preparation for the next world. The discovery of remarkably well-preserved mummies up to 5000 years after their preparation is a tribute to the embalmer's art.

By around 3000 BC priests who had been using the oils in religious ceremonies and embalming rites became aware of the usefulness of their properties for the living, too. Closely guarding their secrets, they became the healers of their time, mixing and prescribing "magic" medicinal potions. Use of essential oils gradually permeated all levels of society as cosmetics and perfumes became widespread.

From Hippocrates we know the Greeks had some awareness of the therapeutic properties of the oils and their value as sedatives and stimulants was certainly recognized. The Greeks and Romans used aromatics widely in rituals and ceremonies and the oils played an important role in the rise in popularity of baths and massage and body-culture generally. However, with the fall of the Roman Empire the use of essential oils died out in Europe.

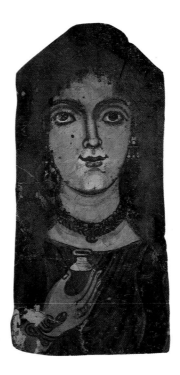

Left: The personal use of perfume was widespread in ancient Greece and Rome. The Roman girl in this portrait (from around AD 350) carries a small pot of aromatics.

Right: From the tomb of the Noble Senedjem, ancient Egypt. The cones of unguent worn on the heads melted in the heat, waxing and scenting the hair and body.

This Milesian container for perfumed oils is fashioned in the form of a Siren, a sea nymph of Greek mythology. It dates from around 525 BC, when Miletus was one of the principal Ionian seaports.

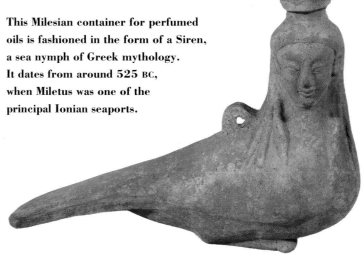

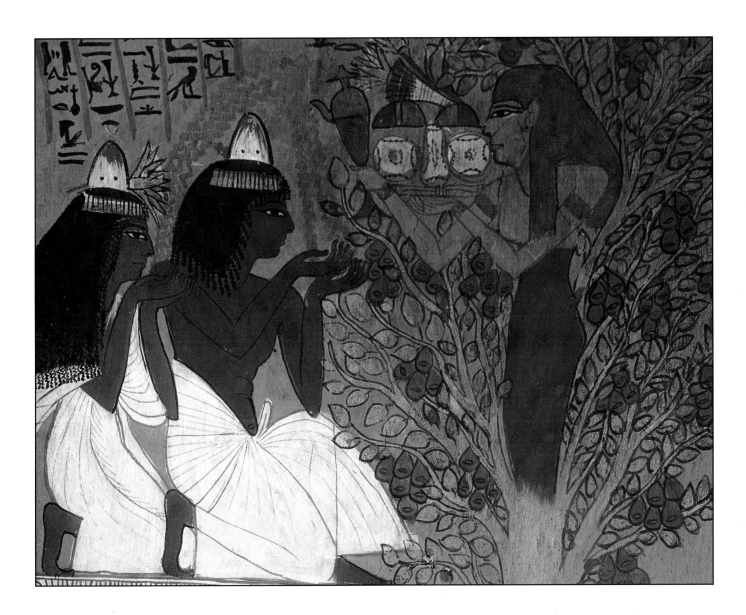

The art flourished elsewhere, though, particularly in Arabia, where Avicenna was the first to distill rose essence around AD 1000. Arabia became the world's centre for production of perfume, importing raw materials from Egypt, India, Tibet and China, and trading their products internationally.

With the Crusaders the art of perfumery was reintroduced to Europe around the twelfth century. Records show that aromatics were used as protection against the plague and the lower incidence of death among perfumiers suggests they were to some degree effective. The fifteenth century saw the rise of the great European perfumiers, and their wares were widely used to disguise body smells and ward off sickness. By the seventeenth century the aphrodisiac properties were certainly well recognized, and with the work of the great herbalists, such as Culpeper, the therapeutic properties also started to be recorded, laying the foundation for modern-day aromatherapy.

THE MODERN RENAISSANCE

The term "Aromathérapie" was first used in 1928 by a French chemist, René-Maurice Gattefossé, to describe the therapeutic action of aromatic plant essences. His work was taken up by Dr Jean Valnet who found the essences' remarkable regenerative and antiseptic properties effective for healing the wounds of World War II soldiers.

The application of aromatherapy to beauty therapy and health care was pioneered by Marguerite Maury in her influential book, *The Secret of Life and Youth*. She also developed the method of applying the oils through massage.

Today there is a world-wide revival in the art of aromatherapy and contemporary research is beginning to understand the scientific foundations of the oils' properties and applications, discovered by trial and error over thousands of years.

ESSENTIAL OILS

The vital element in any aromatherapy treatment is the pure essential oil. These oils are very different from the heavy oils we use for cooking; they are· concentrated essences, much lighter than water and highly flammable. They evaporate quickly, so they are usually mixed with other ingredients to trap their effectiveness. Because they are so concentrated, essential oils are measured in drops.

ESSENCE

This is a natural living substance: the "living" element of a plant which is captured and capsuled. It is a delicate operation. For instance, certain petals and leaves must be picked at exactly the right moment, or the quality of the oil is affected. Only the purest essences are used in aromatherapy so that the therapeutic properties are maximized and the effects are predictable.

Essential oils are extracted from an array of plant sources – petals, leaves, seeds, nut kernels, bark, stalks, flower heads and gums and resins from trees. Apart from their sensuous vapours, which provide the fragrance in many perfumes, they can be used in the bath, smoothed over the body, and used in the myriad ways described in this book.

Because of their small molecular structure, essential oils can penetrate the skin more effectively than vegetable oils, which only lie on the surface. Used medicinally over the centuries, essential oils have now become an established "alternative" natural therapy which can assist in the treatment of almost every type of ache and pain, as well as smoothing away the stress and strains of modern life.

HOW THEY WORK

Essential oils are composed of tiny molecules which are easily dissolved in alcohol, emulsifiers and, particularly, fats. This allows them to penetrate the skin easily and work into the body by mixing with the fatty tissue.

As these highly volatile essences evaporate they are also inhaled, thus entering the body via the millions of sensitive cells that line the nasal passages. These send messages straight to the brain, and affect the emotions by working on the limbic system, which also controls the major functions of the body. Thus in an aromatherapy treatment the essential oils are able to enhance both your physical and psychological well-being at the same time.

Each oil has a distinct chemical composition which determines its fragrance, colour, volatility and, of course, the ways in which it affects the system, giving each oil its unique set of beneficial properties.

METHODS OF EXTRACTION

Distillation
The Egyptians stored their raw materials in large clay or alabaster pots. Water was added and the pots

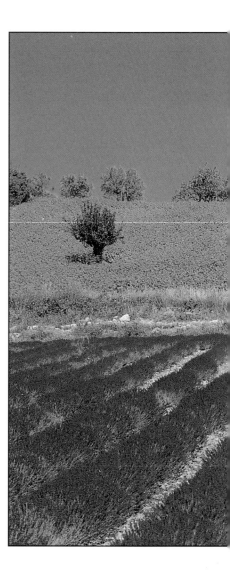

Main picture: Field of lavender, Drome, southern France. French lavender produces the finest quality oil, with a fruitier and sweeter aroma than English lavender, which has a camphorous undertone. It takes one ton (one tonne) of plants to yield about 20 lb (9 kg) of essential oils.

Inset top: Egyptian relief showing perfume-making, from the fourth century BC. The large alabaster pot (a "linge") was filled with flowers, herbs and water, and then heated. The aromatic vapours would saturate a cloth stretched across the pot's opening.

Inset below: Art meets science in the skills of the perfumier, blending a subtle new fragrance from the hundreds of essential oils at his disposal.

heated so that steam rose and was pushed through a cotton cloth in the neck of the jar. This soaked up the essential oil which was then squeezed and pressed out into a collection vessel. The same principle remains in use today as high-pressure steam is passed over the leaves or flowers in a sophisticated still often using a vacuum, so that the essential oils within them vaporize. When the steam carrying the essential oil passes through a cooling system, the oil condenses and can be separated easily from the water.

Maceration
Flowers are soaked in hot oil to break down the cells, releasing their fragrance into the oil which is then purified and the aromatics extracted.

Enfleurage
This is the method by which flower essences, such as jasmine, neroli and rose, which are more delicate and difficult to obtain, are extracted. Flowers or petals are crushed between wooden-framed, glass trays smeared with a greasy animal fat until the fat is saturated with their perfume.

Pressing
This is a simple method of squeezing out, literally, essential oils from the rinds and peel of ripe fruit, such as orange and lemon, into a sponge.

QUALITY CONTROL

Once the flowers and plants are harvested they are usually processed and stored quickly to preserve the freshness. Climate, soil and altitude can all affect the character of an oil. French lavender, for example, is famous for its rich aroma but, like wine, the quality can vary from year to year.

Always buy pure and natural essential oils as synthetic clones or adulterated oils do not act on the body in the same way and many of the beneficial properties are lost. The best quality oils may be expensive but they are always worth the extra cost.

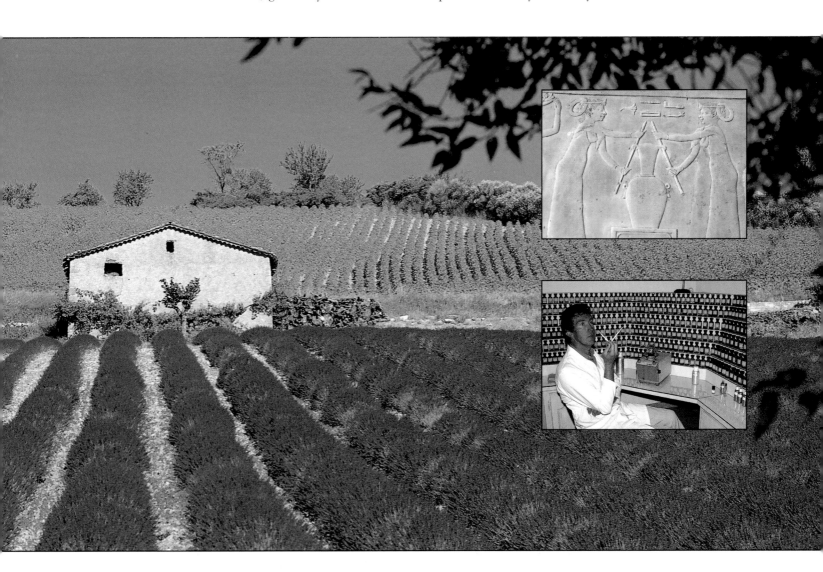

USING ESSENTIAL OILS

You can soak and splash in them, feed your skin, sensually smooth them all over, or simply breathe in their wonderful aromas. The pleasure and versatility of aromatic oils make them one of nature's kindest gifts. Essential oils contain the active ingredients of a plant in a highly concentrated and potent form. They therefore need to be treated with care and should never be applied directly to the skin undiluted. However, there are many ways of dispersing their fragrance and utilizing their therapeutic properties, and most methods do not require any special equipment.

Inhalation
Steam inhalation is an excellent method for treating respiratory problems, colds and so forth, but should not be used by asthmatics. Add 6–12 drops to a bowl of steaming hot water. Place a towel over your head and breathe deeply. This is also a great way of deep-cleansing the face.

Therapeutic Massage
This is the classic aromatherapy treatment, triggering the body's natural healing process by using lymphatic massage and essential oils to stimulate the flow of blood and lymph fluid. The aromas also act upon the emotional centre in the brain (the "limbic" system) which governs the way we feel.
For massage use a 1–3 per cent solution of essential oil to base oil.

Fragrancers
These attractive pots, also known as diffusers or vaporizers, are simple to use. Fill the top china bowl with water and add a few drops of essential oil on to the surface. The candle in the pot underneath heats the water, slowly releasing the natural fragrance of the oil into the room.
Stand the burner on a plate or tile, not on plastic surfaces.

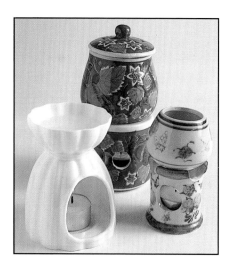

Decorative fragancers for diffusing essential oils.

3–6 drops of essential oil are sufficient, depending on the size of the room. It is also possible to buy battery-driven fan vaporizers which blow air through oil-impregnated pads, which can be changed to suit the mood.

Baths
Run hand-hot water and then add 5–10 drops of the essential oil to suit your mood. Close the door, keep in the vapours, and soak for 15 minutes. For sensitive skin it is better to dilute the oil in a base oil first, like sweet almond, apricot or peach kernel. Essential oils can mark plastic baths if they are not dispersed thoroughly. Wipe the bath straight after use.

Foot Bath
Refresh tired feet by adding 4–5 drops of peppermint, rosemary and thyme to a large bowl of hot water. Soothe with lavender.

Hand Bath
Soothe chapped skin by soaking in bowl of warm water (not hot) with 3–4 drops of patchouli or comfrey before a manicure.

Shower
After soaping or gelling, rinse well. Dip a wet sponge in an oil mix of your choice, squeeze and rub over your whole body while under a warm jet spray.

Sauna
Add two drops of eucalyptus or pine oil per $\frac{1}{2}$ pint (330 ml) of water and throw over the coals to evaporate. These are great cleansers and detoxifiers.

Jacuzzi or Hot Tub
Relax by adding 10–15 drops of sandalwood, geranium or ylang-ylang, or simply bubble over with the stimulating effects of pine, rosemary and neroli.

Room Sprays

To make a room spray blend ten drops of essential oil in seven tablespoons of water. One tablespoon of vodka or pure alcohol added to the solution will act as a preservative but this is optional. Shake well before filling the sprayer.

Pillow Talk

Perfume your pillow with 2–3 drops of oil. Choose a relaxing oil to unwind or one for insomnia if you have sleep problems. For a different mood, try an aphrodisiac like ylang-ylang or be extravagant and use rose or jasmine, the two most expensive pure oils.

Perfumes

The finest perfumes are traditionally blended from pure essential oils, particularly the flower extracts, though these days synthetic aromas tend to be used, particularly for cheaper perfumes. The art of the perfumier is subtle and skilled, and difficult to emulate at home as it is hard to find a medium to use as a substitute for alcohol. If you have a favourite oil or blend of essences you can use it all over in a body oil (three per cent solution); or make a very concentrated blend (25 per cent) to dab behind ears, knees and on wrists and temples.

Pomanders

Hang porous corked bottles in the wardrobe. The essential oil is absorbed by the clay and released slowly. Fill with the fragrance of your choice: try melissa or bergamot, or cedarwood to keep away moths.

Pot Pourri

Add a few drops of an appropriate flowery or spicy essential oil to refresh tired pot pourri, or make your own.

Handkerchief

The most portable way of using essential oils. Add 3–4 drops to a handkerchief and inhale. Useful for treating colds or headaches, or for clearing your head at work.

Shoe Rack

Freshen the cupboard with lemongrass. Deodorize shoes with two drops of pine or parsley oil.

From the top: perfume bottle, pot pourri and oil lamp.

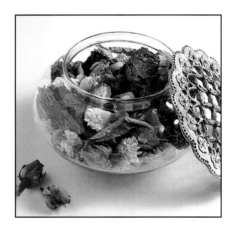

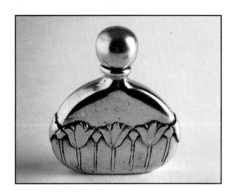

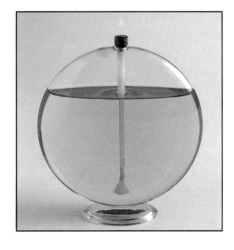

Humidifiers

You can add your favourite oil to the water of a humidifier or improvize by adding five drops of essential oil to a small bowl of water placed on top of a radiator.

Ring Burners

Use the heat from light bulbs to release perfumed oils. Small ring burners, usually made of porcelain or aluminium, sit over the top of the bulb. Add a few drops of essential oil, and the heat from the bulb will gently vaporize the essential oil.

Wood Fires

Sprinkle drops of cypress, cedarwood, pine or sandalwood over the logs to be used about an hour before lighting the fire and then burn them to release your favourite aroma.

Scented Candles

Wax candles can be bought ready-impregnated with essential oils and are a delightful way of fragrancing a room. Or you can add a few drops of essential oil to an oil lamp for the same effect.

Compresses

Soak a clean cotton cloth (such as a face flannel, handkerchief or small towel) in $\frac{1}{4}$ pint (160 ml) warm water with 5–10 drops of essential oil. Squeeze out and lay across the area to be treated. Cover and leave until cold. A useful method for sprains, bruising, headaches (place the compress across the forehead) and hot flushes.

Body and Facial Oils

These can be used on a daily basis to nourish the skin. Use a one per cent blend of essential oil to carrier oil for the face and a three per cent blend for the body.

BLENDING AND STORING

Essential oils are the basis for all traditional aromatherapy. Each one has a particular fragrance and properties and the art of blending them harmoniously combines the skills of the perfumier and the pharmacist. Although two essences may have a similar smell or property they may not necessarily mix well together. One essence can overpower the other. For example, frankincense and ginger, both heavy smelling essences, give an overpowering, unpleasant smell when combined, whereas lavender and rosemary happily marry together. In general it is best to use a maximum of three oils in a blend so there is less chance of detracting from their individual qualities.

Assemble bottles of different sizes for storing appropriate quantities of blended oils. Funnels and droppers ensure accurate measurements and help prevent spillages.

THE ART OF BLENDING

Essential oils are highly volatile substances which should be handled, mixed and stored with care and used sparingly. Spillage of one particular oil can overpower a whole room and adversely affect young children and animals.

The power of aromatics is quite subtle. Never try to sniff or smell a pure essential oil straight from the bottle. Place a drop on the side of a glass and become a connoisseur: sniff, consider and take notes if you wish.

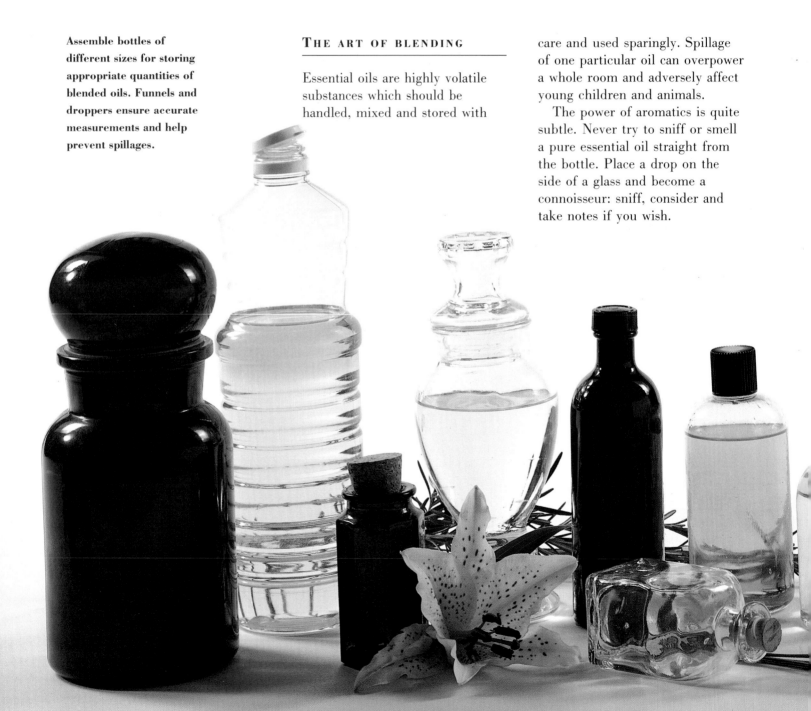

MIXING

Base oils play an important role in carrying and diluting highly concentrated essential oils, which are only used in small quantities measured in drops. These base oils dilute the pure essentials, inhibiting the evaporation rate and – since they spread evenly and easily over skin – encouraging quick absorption of the therapeutic oils into the skin.

When mixing, use a glass, porcelain or aluminium bottle and check that you have the correct amount of vegetable carrier oil before adding the recommended drops of essentials with a dropper or pipette for accurate measurements. Mix well and label the bottles clearly.

If you accidentally spill any, wipe up instantly with a paper tissue and dispose of it outside as the smell will be overpowering.

STORING

Dark glass bottles with stoppered caps are used to store essential oils. At home, keep them in a cool dark place, stand them upright, and always out of sight and touch of children. Never store essential oils in plastic bottles: both the oil and the bottle will perish. Oils will keep for at least a year if properly stored, although citrus oils may have a shorter life.

CARRIER OILS

ase oils are normally extracted from nuts or seeds and each has its own particular quality. Sweet almond oil is probably the best all-purpose carrier oil because it is neutral and non-allergenic. It can even be used for massaging babies. Walnut acts as a co-ordinator and balances the nervous system; sesame is ideal for stretch marks; apricot kernel, peach kernel and evening primrose oils are all good for cell regeneration. Walnut and evening primrose oil help alleviate menstrual problems including pre-menstrual tension. Wheatgerm acts as an anti-oxidant and will help preserve a mixture.

These oils are all rich in nutrients, and are ideal for most dry and sensitive skin types. The most important thing when buying these basics is to check that they have been naturally processed and not chemically treated. Cold-pressed is best.

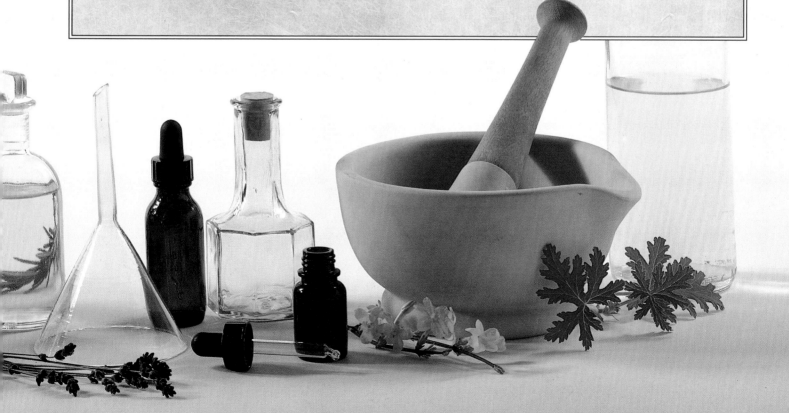

AROMATICS

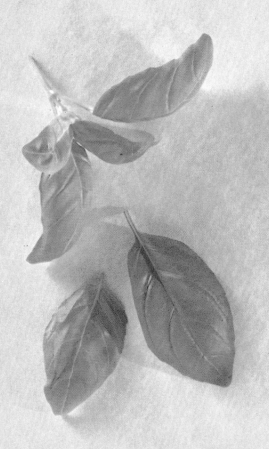

Aromatic oils extracted from flowers, fruits, leaves, barks, resins and roots have been used throughout the centuries for their healing properties and marvellous fragrances. Hundreds of essential oils are used today in such industries as food, cosmetics, pharmaceuticals and perfumery. Modern-day aromatherapy uses a much smaller selection, but the range of aromas and applications is nonetheless remarkable.

This section is a connoisseurs' guide to thirty-five of the most popular, versatile and safe oils. Get to know their individual characters, their origins, their therapeutic values and discover your own favourites. Lavender, geranium and rosemary are excellent all-round oils and provide a good basis for any collection. Rose, though expensive, is also well worth the investment if you would like to explore the benefits and delights of aromatherapy.

BASIL

Ocimum basilicum

Origins Basil was used in baths and body massage by ancient Greek nobles for its fragrant perfume. The Egyptians used the aromatic fragrance in their offerings to the gods and also mixed it with essences of myrrh and incense to embalm bodies. In India it is believed to offer protection to the soul and is sacred to the Hindu gods Krishna and Vishnu.

Description Native of Africa and the Seychelles and now grown as a popular culinary herb in Europe, it can grow up to three feet (90 cm) in height and has small white flowers. The essence is distilled from the leaves and is a light greenish-yellow with sweet green overtones.

Therapeutic effects Ideal as a nerve tonic, to lift fatigue, anxiety and depression. Also good for bronchitis, colds, fever, gout and indigestion, and reputed to soothe snake bites.

Uses Inhalation, baths and massage. It has both hot and cold qualities. When used in the bath or smoothed over the body it has an invigorating effect – great for sluggish skin and pepping up circulation. Combined with other oils such as thyme it also acts as a powerful antiseptic.

Cautionary note A powerful depressant if over-used. Also best to avoid during pregnancy.

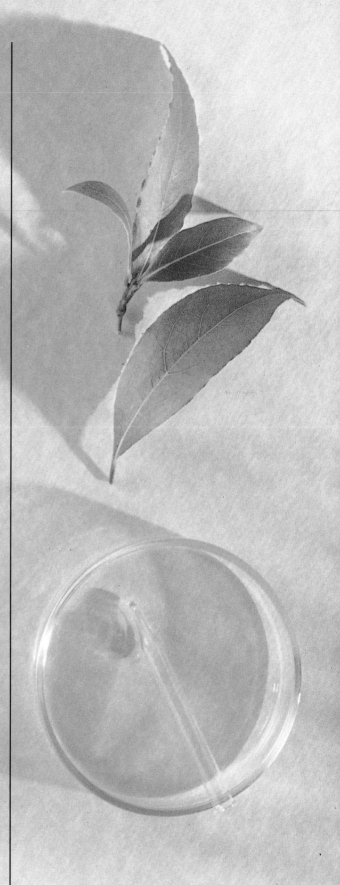

BAY

Pimenta racemosa

Origins Roman emperors wore sprigs of bay, known as *Laurus nobilis* (Roman laurel), not only as a sign of wealth, but to ward off evil spirits. Greek priestesses chewed the leaves for their soporific effect, and after gastronomic banquets it was chewed as a breath freshener.

Description Popular as a culinary herb, bay is an attractive evergreen shrub whose shiny leathery leaves produce clusters of yellowish-green flowers in spring. The spicy-smelling oil is extracted from the leaves and is yellowish-brown in colour.

Therapeutic effects As a pulmonary antiseptic, it helps relieve bronchitis, colds and flu. Also used to aid digestion and sleep, to soothe rheumatic aches and pains, and as a general tonic.

Uses Inhalation, baths and massage. Widely used in perfume and exotic bath essences for its uplifting effects.

BENZOIN

Styrax benzoin

Origins In the Far East the gum from the benzoin tree was one of the main ingredients used in incense to drive away evil spirits. The compound tincture is highly potent, pharmaceutically used in friar's balsam and as a fixative in perfume.

Description The benzoin tree is cultivated in Borneo, Java, Malaysia, Sumatra and Thailand. Like the rubber tree, its gum is taken from the bark by making a deep incision in the trunk. The gum is dark, with reddish-brown coloured streaks. These pigments contain the fatty oils which exude a delicious aroma similar to vanilla.

Therapeutic effects Valuable for treating urinary infections, it has a warming, relaxing, action suitable for respiratory conditions such as bronchitis, coughs and colds. Also effective for relieving skin conditions, and for gout.

Uses Inhalation, massage and in cough medicines. This is an energizing oil which can be used in one of two forms: simple tincture or compound – the former is not so toxic and is preferable for skin conditions.

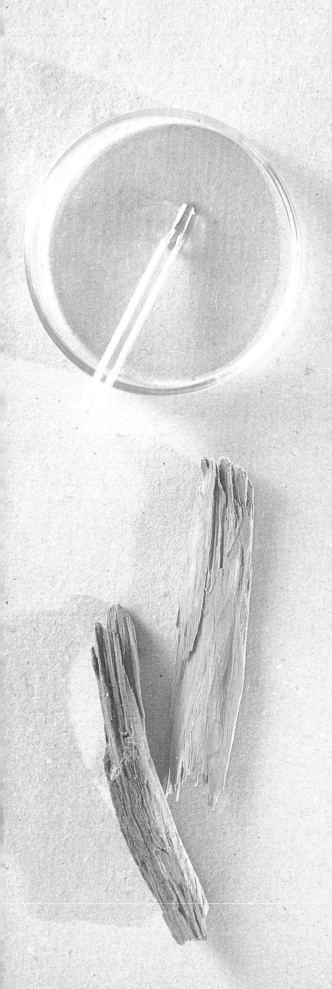

BERGAMOT
Citrus bergamia

Origins Native to Morocco, it wasn't until bergamot rooted in Italy that its essential properties were recognized.

Description The bergamot tree belongs to the same family as the orange tree and the essential oil, as in most citrus varieties, is expressed from the fresh peel of the fruit. The oil is emerald green in colour, and smells spicier than lemon but with a similar, citrus quality. The odour is familiar from its use as a flavouring in Earl Grey tea.

Therapeutic effects Has a powerful uplifting and refreshing action. As an antiseptic it has proved effective in the treatment of mouth and skin infections, and sore throats. Can lower fever, and help with bronchitis and indigestion.

Uses Bergamot blends well with most essences and is a popular top note in perfumery. Along with neroli and lavender it is a main ingredient in eau-de-Cologne and is commonly used in toiletries to refresh and relax. In massage it can stimulate or soothe depending on the oils with which it is mixed.

Cautionary note In concentrations above one per cent it can irritate the skin. Also, even though it is sometimes added to commercial suntan agents to stimulate melanin production, it must never be used in home mixtures for tanning purposes.

CEDARWOOD
Juniperus virginiana

Origins Cedarwood oil, similar to sandalwood, was used by the Egyptians in the embalming process. It was highly prized for its antiseptic properties and so became an important ingredient in cosmetics. Originally it was made from the beautiful Lebanon cedar, but, over-felled for furniture, this is now very scarce, and the red cedar is primarily used in its place.

Description The cedar is grown in North Africa and the USA for its highly valued, fragrant wood. The clear, syrupy essential oil is extracted by steam distillation of waste woods. The odour of the oil is reminiscent of wooden pencils.

Therapeutic effects Used for skin complaints such as acne, alopecia, dandruff and eczema, and respiratory problems, especially bronchitis and catarrh. Also acts as a diuretic for help in urinary infections.

Uses Inhalation and massage. Increases sexual response. Blends well with cypress, juniper and rose.

Cautionary note Will irritate the skin in high concentrations.

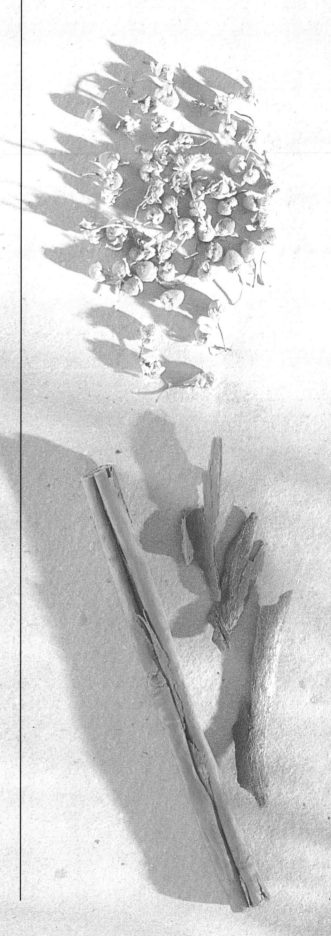

CHAMOMILE
Alternative spelling: Camomile
Anthemis nobilis

Origins The Egyptians thought this was a sacred flower and dedicated it to the Sun God. It was used in ritual ceremonies and medicinally to stop fits and fevers.

Description Chamomile species grow throughout Europe, North Africa and are often found growing wild. They have fine, feathery leaves with tiny white or yellow-centred daisy-like flowers. The pale blue oil is extracted from the flower and has a slightly apple fragrance which blends well with rose, geranium and lavender.

Therapeutic effects Particularly noted for its anti-inflammatory and sedative properties, it is excellent for childhood ailments (whether in children or adults!) from peevishness to earache. Also used for allergies, anaemia, burns, dermatitis, diarrhoea, fever, indigestion, insomnia, menstrual and menopausal problems, rheumatism, toothache and ulcers.

Uses Certain chamomile species are used for herbal infusions, but the oil is used in body, bath and hair products for its anti-allergenic properties. Use in dilute form for children.

CINNAMON
Cinnamomum zeylanicum

Origins The Chinese believed that no remedy or treatment was complete without cinnamon. It is one of the oldest spices known – used by the Egyptians, Romans and Greeks, and it was also mentioned in the Old Testament.

Description Grown in the Far East, East Indies, and China, cinnamon has a distinctive hot, peppery aroma and taste. The twigs and leaves are picked and distilled to produce a sweet, pungent and bitter aromatic oil, which is a dark yellow-brown in colour. Its warm, spicy essence is often used in perfumery.

Therapeutic effects Useful for fatigue and depression, it is also a tonic for the respiratory and digestive systems, especially useful for coughs, colds, flu, stomach ache and diarrhoea. An aphrodisiac, it may also help impotence.

Uses Inhalation and massage. Burn to prevent the spread of flu virus, or add bark or oil to spice up a pot pourri. To relieve muscular spasms use in a compress or massage.

Cautionary note Use only in very low concentrations or under professional advice.

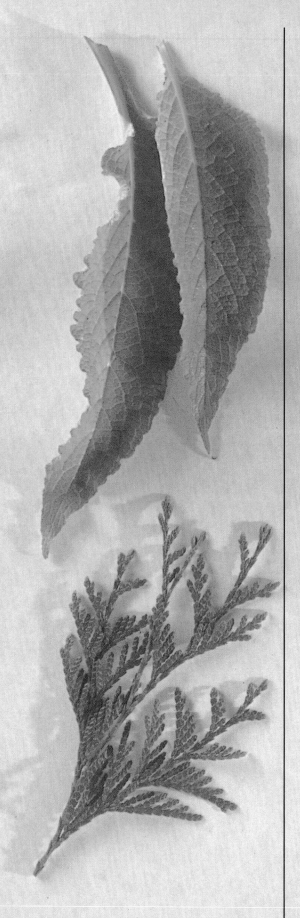

COMFREY

Symphtum officinale

Origins Herbalist Nicholas Culpeper wrote in his medicinal scripts in the seventeenth century that this herb 'helpeth those that spit blood or make a bloody urine'. The root boiled in water or wine was drunk to help solve all internal problems, inwardly healing wounds, ulcers of the lungs and to help the flow of blood.

Description Normally grows wild near damp watersides. Comfrey has large hairy leaves which can irritate the skin if touched. The stalk grows to three feet (90 cm) high with pale purplish flowers. The leaves and roots are used in herbal decoctions but the oil is extracted from the leaves and stalks.

Therapeutic effects Containing allantoin, a cell regenerator, comfrey oil is particularly valuable for the treatment of wounds and skin disorders, including eczema, psoriasis, athlete's foot and torn muscles. Helpful, too, in treating stretch marks and for menopausal and menstrual problems.

Uses Massage and compresses.

CYPRESS

Cupressus sempervirens

Origins Egyptians used this wood to adorn their stone coffins along with using the oil for its medicinal properties. In France it is traditionally planted in graveyards.

Description A tall, conical, evergreen tree, it originated in the East but is popularly grown throughout the Mediterranean area, especially in Algeria and southern France. The essence is obtained by the distillation of the leaves, twigs and cones of the tree. Clear, pale yellow or green, it has a refreshing, spicy fragrance, reminiscent of pine-needles.

Therapeutic effects Most noted for its astringent and antispasmodic qualities, it can be used for circulatory conditions, colds, coughs, flu, haemorrhoids, menstrual and menopausal problems, varicose veins and whooping cough. It also acts as a sedative to soothe nervous tension.

Uses Inhalation, baths and massage. Use in compresses for swelling or rheumatism or in the bath as a muscular tonic. Its astringent properties make it suitable for use in cleansers for oily skin.

Cautionary note Not to be used by anyone who suffers from high blood pressure.

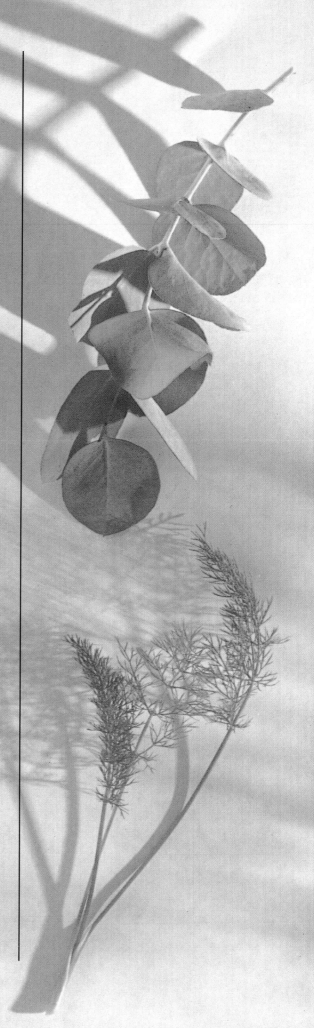

EUCALYPTUS

Eucalyptus globulus

Origins One of the tallest trees in the world, it originated in Australia and later grew in Tasmania, China, USA, Brazil and the Mediterranean. There are something like 200 species. The Aborigines may have been the first to use it medicinally.

Description The silvery, blue–green leaves produce a pale yellow oil which has a cool, camphorous smell. The fresh leaves give a rich yield of highly potent essence, one of the most versatile in aromatherapy.

Therapeutic effects The principal constituent of the oil is the antiseptic eucalyptol. Combined with its anti-inflammatory properties, eucalyptus oil is particularly helpful for asthma, bronchitis, flu, sinusitis, skin infections, rheumatism and sores. It can also reduce fever, is a strong diuretic, and its head-clearing qualities are well-known.

Uses Baths, inhalation and massage. It has a cooling effect on body temperature, reduces fever and is also a remedy for muscular/rheumatic aches and pains. It is widely used in cold and cough medicines and rubs. Use in the bath to relieve cystitis or on a handkerchief to clear the head.

FENNEL

Foeniculum vulgare

Origins The ancient Greeks and Romans advocated the strongly flavoured fennel seeds to give them strength, to ward off evil spirits, kill fleas, and sweeten the breath.

Description These graceful perennial plants are found in Europe, often by the sea, and have delicate bright green feathery foliage. Their bright tufts of yellow flowers attract the bees. As a herb, the fresh leaves are particularly valued for fish dishes whereas the seeds, which smell like aniseed, are used in liquorice. The sweet oil, which has a similar smell, is extracted from the crushed seeds.

Therapeutic effects Noted as a diuretic, and a mild laxative, fennel has been found effective for colic, constipation, digestive problems, kidney stones, menopausal problems, nausea and obesity. It is also often helpful for increasing milk yield during breast feeding.

Uses Massage. The sweet aromatic oil is mainly used for flavouring medicines to help flatulence and indigestion. It is a constituent of gripe water, and can be infused in teas.

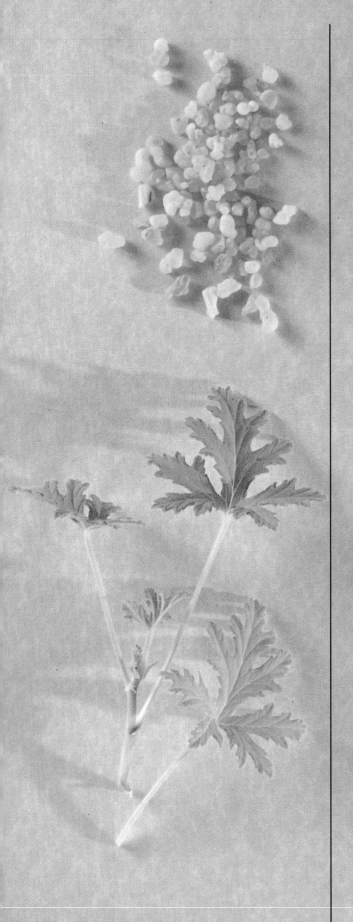

FRANKINCENSE
Boswellia thurifera

Origins Frankincense (also known as olibanum) and myrrh were the first tree resins used as incense by the Egyptians. They were burned to clear the air in sickrooms and during religious ceremonies to drive away evil spirits. They ranked alongside precious stones as a valuable commodity and, according to the Bible, were offered by the three Kings to celebrate the birth of Jesus Christ. The gum comes from a small tree grown in Arabia, Africa, and China. It was first brought to Europe in the late seventeenth century.

Description To make the gum a deep incision is made in the tree trunk where the resin exudes in tear-shaped globules which harden on contact with air. The essence is spicy, with camphor undertones, but becomes lemony when mixed with myrrh.

Therapeutic effects Has an uplifting effect and aids concentration. Helpful as an expectorant in cases of bronchitis, coughs, colds and laryngitis. Reputed to preserve a youthful skin, eradicating wrinkles.

Uses Inhalation, baths and massage. Inhale to release catarrh, or relax with a few drops in a bath or body massage oil to warm, relax and meditate. It is often combined with myrrh, and blends well with essences such as basil and sandalwood.

GERANIUM
Pelargonium adorantissimum

Origins The geranium originates in Africa and was not brought into Europe until 1690. It was used in ancient times as a remedy for tumours, burns and wounds.

Description Widely grown throughout Europe, it reaches around two feet (60 cm) in height. There are hundreds of different species cultivated for their pretty flowers, but only the aromatic pelargoniums (the ones that smell lemony when the leaves are pinched) give rich yields of the sweet yellowy-green essential oil. This is distilled from the leaves, stalks and flowers.

Therapeutic effects Unusually, it is both sedative and uplifting, and so invaluable for treating nervous tension and depression. Also used for circulatory and skin problems, especially wounds. Use in a footbath for chilblains.

Uses All uses. A popular ingredient in perfumes for its sweet, fresh, floral essence, the geranium is also therapeutically massaged or inhaled for its relaxing yet refreshing qualities. It can blend well with most other essential oils.

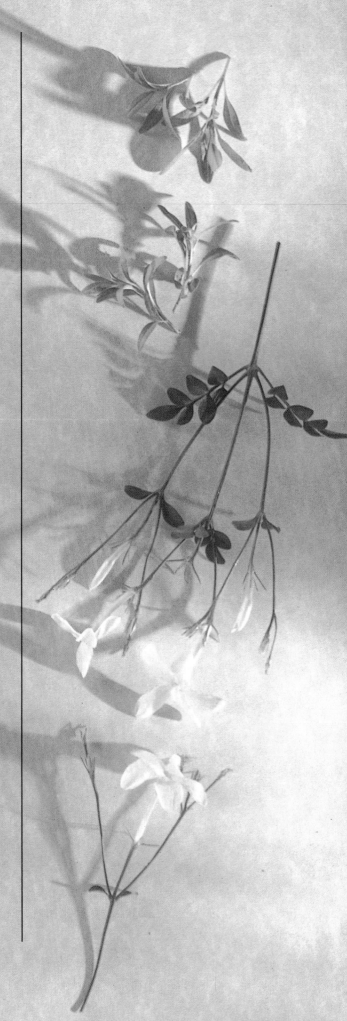

HYSSOP

Hyssopus officinalis

Origins Ancient alchemists used the powdered leaves and roots as a purgative and in ointments to spread over the stomach to combat worms. Small doses taken internally were mixed with honey to clean the mucous matter from the intestines or with crushed figs to loosen the bowels.

Description A small herbal perennial, hyssop has long stalks with narrow leaves and blue flowers. The oil, extracted from the leaves and flowering heads, is used in perfumes and liqueurs, including Chartreuse.

Therapeutic effects Hyssop is used for disorders of the cardiovascular system, and as it is both stimulating and sedative, it can regulate blood pressure whether high or low. It has powerful effects on the respiratory tract, for bronchitis, coughs and colds, and is also used for skin disorders.

Uses Massage and inhalation. It is also used in cough mixtures for bronchial conditions.

Cautionary note Use only in extremely small quantities. Do not use during pregnancy.

JASMINE

Jasminum officinale

Origins An ancient favourite of the Arabs, Indians and Chinese, jasmine had a wide variety of uses including perfuming the body, scenting rooms and flavouring herbal teas. It was introduced from Persia to Europe in the sixteenth century.

Description The *Jasminum grandiflora* species is a small bush, native to the East Indies and Egypt and cultivated in southern France, Spain, Algeria, Morocco, India and Egypt. Its delicate white flowers produce a honey-sweet floral bouquet with fruity undertones. The deep red oil is produced by *enfleurage*, and has an intense rich, floral fragrance that is warm and exotic. It is one of the most important and expensive extracts, along with rose, used in perfumery.

Therapeutic effects Jasmine is a mood enhancer, lifting anxiety and depression. An aphrodisiac, it has a reputation for the treatment of both frigidity and impotence. It will also relieve menstrual cramps and is soothing to inflamed or irritated skin.

Uses Inhalation, bathing and massage will all exploit its warming and relaxing qualities. Also makes a delightful uplifting perfume or room fragrance.

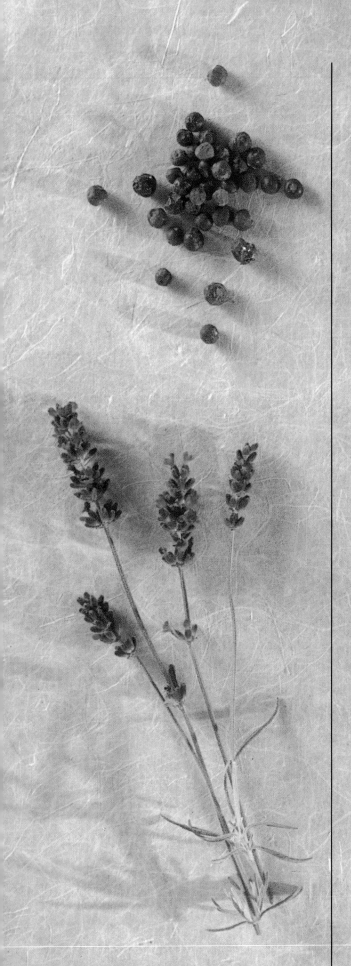

JUNIPER
Juniperus communis

Origins Grown in North America, Asia, Africa and Europe, this small shrub with aromatic leaves and berries was popular as incense to burn in religious ceremonies and to purify the air and ward off the plague.

Description An evergreen bush with thick branches and narrow needle leaves, juniper produces small yellow flowers and small purplish-blue berries. Both the berries and leaves have a strong aromatic fragrance, similar to pine-needles, but the oil is extracted from the berries by distillation, producing a pale yellow essence.

Therapeutic effects Diuretic and antiseptic, it is especially effective for the urinary tract and an excellent treatment for cystitis and water retention. Use for acne, colic, coughs, dermatitis, eczema, flatulence, rheumatism and skin ulcers.

Uses Inhalation, baths and massage. The oil is a great stimulator and, like cypress and pine, makes a refreshing bath oil. Massaged on the skin it stimulates the circulation.

LAVENDER
Lavendula officinalis

Origins Lavender comes from the Roman word "lavare" meaning to wash. It was one of most favoured aromatics used by the Romans in their daily bathing rituals. Both the Greeks and Romans burned lavender twigs as a room purifier to ward off the plague. It was brought to Europe by the Romans.

Description A shrubby plant with woody branches and long narrow leaves, it has purple-blue flowers on long spikes. After cutting, the plants are dried and steam-distilled. The essential oil is clear to pale yellow in colour with a strong aroma.

Therapeutic effects Its sedative and tonic effects make lavender a great balancer of the nervous and emotional systems. Excellent for migraine. As an antiseptic it can be used for many skin conditions and infections of the lungs, digestion and unrinary tract. Extraordinarily versatile.

Uses Inhalation, baths, room spray, massage and most other uses. Use as a cold compress or place a few drops in boiling water and inhale for headaches and migraine. A warm towel wrap will soothe nervous exhaustion. A late-night lavender bath will help combat sleeplessness.

LEMON

Citrus limonum

Origins Early seafarers stocked up with fresh lemons before a long voyage to help prevent scurvy and to purify the ship's drinking water. Its astringent and antiseptic properties were fully appreciated in the first aid kit and used to treat cuts, bruises and insect stings.

Description The lemon tree, which has white–pink flowers and bright yellow fruits, is cultivated in most Mediterranean countries, Brazil, USA, Argentina, Israel and Africa. The pale yellow oil is expressed from the rind and peel of the fruit and has classically been used in perfume for its intense, sharp, citrus-fresh aroma. The essence becomes cloudy, and deteriorates over time, if not properly stored.

Therapeutic effects Lemon is highly antiseptic and astringent, and so is naturally used for skin complaints including boils, warts and veruccas. Also good for lowering blood pressure, colds, digestive problems, fever and gallstones.

Uses Inhalation, baths and massage. Lemon, as with most citrus oils, is a good cleanser inside and out. Use in skin-care preparations for oily skin. Evaporated in a fragrancer it will help colds and act as an insect repellent.

LEMONGRASS

Cymbopogon citratus

Origins This sweet-scented grass was mainly used to season food in India, the African Congo, the Seychelles, Indonesia and Sri Lanka. Its main constituent, citral, was discovered to be a strong, cleansing antiseptic, and used to deodorize clothing and footwear. Dried leaves were burned to keep the mind alert.

Description Lemongrass is a tall-stemmed, grass-like tropical plant. Its oil is steam-distilled from the fresh or partly dried grasses, and has a refreshing, lemony smell. It is used in low-cost citrus soaps, perfumes and cleaning agents.

Therapeutic effects Through its anti-bacterial action, it is good for skin complaints, sore throats and respiratory problems. Also effective against headaches.

Uses Inhalation and massage. For the active work-out enthusiast, lemongrass is the ideal cooler and deodorizer. It can help alleviate athlete's foot and its refreshing fragrance acts as an energizer. Massaged or breathed in, it tones the heart and works on the digestive system. The oil will also repel insects.

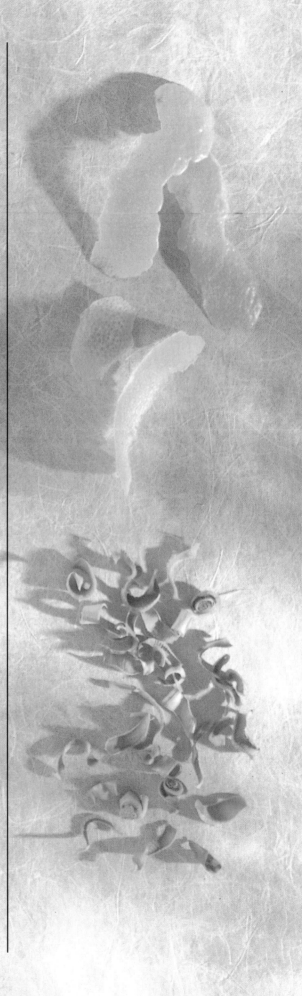

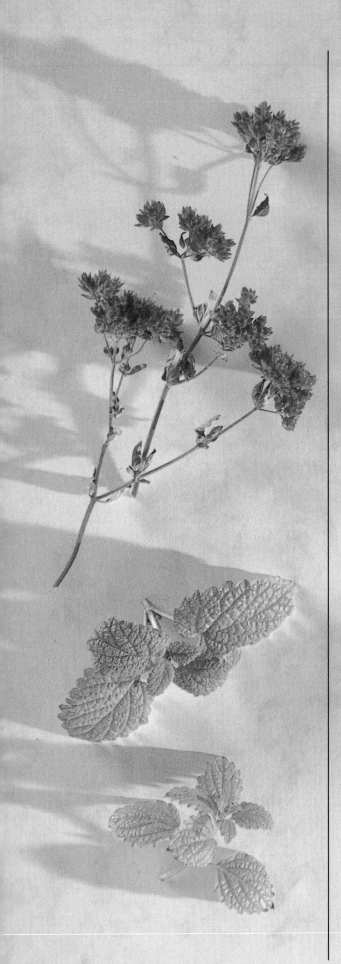

MARJORAM

Origanum marjorana

Origins The Greeks grew marjoram for use in their perfumes and herbal potions. They prescribed it as a medicinal antidote and to purge the system.

Description This popular perennial plant is one of the classic culinary herbs, and is grown world-wide. The amber-coloured essence is extracted by steam-distillation from the fresh and dried leaves and flowering tops. Its warm and slightly spicy aroma is often used in masculine fragrances.

Therapeutic effects A warming agent, able to relieve spasm, it is particularly valuable for treating the nervous system. Use for anxiety and insomnia, but also for arthritis, asthma, bronchitis, circulatory problems, constipation, headaches, menstrual problems, muscular strains and rheumatism.

Uses Inhalation and massage. It blends well with bergamot, lavender and rosemary. In bath and body oils it gives a warm, relaxing feeling. Steam-inhaled or smoothed over the sinuses and temples, it can relieve colds.

Cautionary note Do not use in early pregnancy. Do not use in high doses as it can have a narcotic effect and is also known to curb sexual drive.

MELISSA

Melissa officinalis

Origins The Greeks and Arabs knew the properties of melissa and in the sixteenth century the Swiss physician Paracelsus hailed it as the "elixir of life".

Description Mostly a native of Europe, it is also cultivated in North America. Better known as sweet balm or lemon balm, it is a bushy perennial of the mint family. The aromatic oil smells like lemons and is extracted from the leaves by distillation.

Therapeutic effects Long known as an uplifting and calming cure for "melancholia", its tonic, antispasmodic properties make it effective too in the treatment of allergies, colds, diarrhoea, hypertension, menstrual problems, migraine and stress headaches, nausea and palpitations.

Uses Inhalation, baths and massage. The essential oil helps lower blood pressure and remove tension. Add six drops to the bath water. Melissa calms the body and mind, yet lifts the soul: an oil to dream with.

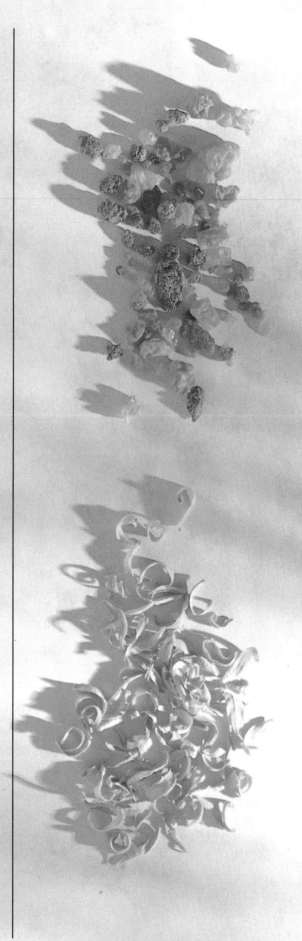

MYRRH

Commiphora myrrha

Origins The Egyptians and the Greeks prized myrrh as a precious commodity. It was used by both civilizations in worshipping their gods, celebration rituals, cosmetics, perfumes and herbal treatments. The Egyptians combined it with frankincense for embalming and purification purposes.

Description A small tree, rather like a bush, myrrh is native in Arabia, Somalia, Ethiopia and other North African countries. Although the leaves are aromatic it is the resin which is distilled to produce the viscous, yellow essential oil. It has a warm, lightly spicy, sweet smell.

Therapeutic effects Anti-inflammatory and expectorant, myrrh will ease bronchitis, catarrh, coughs and colds. Good too for digestive problems, infections of the mouth and throat, and skin conditions.

Uses Inhalation and massage. It is used in pharmaceuticals and perfumery. In aromatherapy, because of its cooling effect, it blends well with camphor and lavender.

NEROLI

Citrus aurantium

Origins Neroli is believed to have been discovered by the Romans. In 1680 it was used to scent the bath water and gloves of Anna Maria Orsini, Princess of Nerola, who brought the fragrance into fashion amongst the Italian aristocracy.

Description Neroli oil is better known as orange blossom. It comes from the white blossoms of the bitter orange tree which originated in China but also grows in Egypt, Morocco, Algeria, USA, Italy and southern France. The pale yellow oil is expensive to produce since it takes approximately one ton (one tonne) of flowers to extract just 2 lb (1 kg) of oil. These are hand picked as they are just about to open and then distilled. Its powerful, wonderfully uplifting, floral fragrance is reminiscent of lilies and is extensively used in eau-de-Cologne.

Therapeutic effects An excellent sedative and anti-depressant, neroli counters anxiety, hysteria, shock and palpitations, and combats insomnia. It is helpful for dermatitis and dry skin, pre-menstrual tension and menopausal problems.

Uses Inhalation, baths and massage. Use in the bath or as a body oil to alleviate the symptoms of pre-menstrual tension and generally improve circulation, or just for the benefits of its delightful fragrance and relaxing properties.

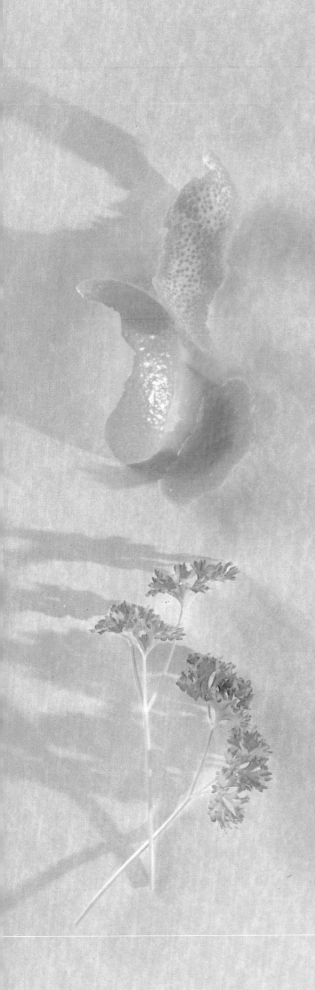

ORANGE

Citrus aurantium (bitter orange),
Citrus sinensis (sweet orange)

Origins China was the first home of the orange tree and the fragrant qualities of sweet and bitter orange oils have long been prized for culinary, cosmetic and medicinal use.

Description The sweet and the bitter oils are similar and both are extracted by cold pressing of fresh orange peel (it is only neroli oil which is extracted from the blossom). The bitter and sweet oils range from yellow to brown in colour and are used extensively for their fresh top notes in perfume.

Therapeutic effects Refreshing but sedative, orange is a tonic for anxiety and depression. It also stimulates the digestive system and is effective for constipation. Its antiseptic properties work well for mouth ulcers.

Uses Baths and massage. These essential oils, rich in vitamin C, are used widely throughout the food and cosmetics industry in products ranging from bath and body oils to chocolate-orange confectionery.

PARSLEY

Petroselinum sativum

Origins A lot of folklore surrounds the parsley plant. It was a medieval belief that it grew in the garden only if the man or woman of the house was "honest". When chewed, it would keep away the devil or, as later discovered, reduce bad breath.

Description Native to Asia Minor, it is now found all over the world. The common parsley is cultivated for its culinary uses and essential oil properties. The highest content of oil comes from the ripe seeds but the leaves are also used in distillation. It has a warm, herbaceous, spicy smell and is used in many herbal perfumes and cosmetic products.

Therapeutic effects A diuretic, useful for kidney and urinary problems and water retention. Also high in vitamin A – essential for healthy hair, skin, teeth and eyes; and iron – for the blood and liver, and during menstruation and menopause.

Uses Massage. It blends well with fennel to help combat excessive water retention when massaged over the body. In conjunction with lemon and rosemary it can help clear toxins in the liver and kidneys. In general, a good oil to help calm the nervous system.

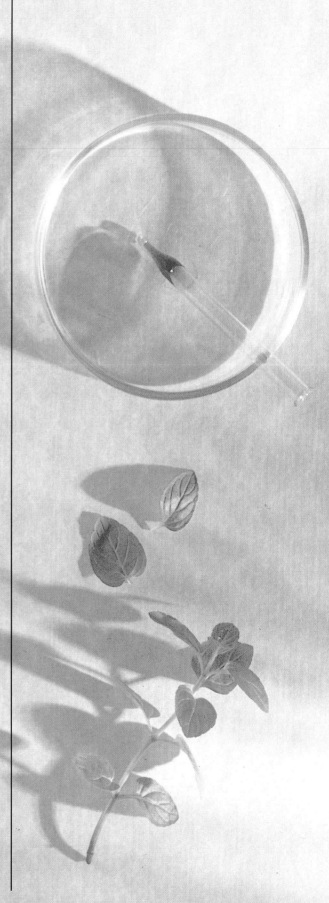

PATCHOULI
Pogostemon patchouli

Origins Along with rose, jasmine, sandalwood and basil, patchouli was one of the favourite perfumes used in India, and shawls and blankets were impregnated with this rich oil. It is an aphrodisiac, and became very popular again in the 1960s for this reason.

Description The oil is extracted from the dried, fermented leaves of the small shrub and emits an intense, woody, sweet-spicy, balsamic odour. It improves with age and is used as a fixative in perfume.

Therapeutic effects Patchouli is an astringent, and is useful for scalp and skin conditions including dandruff, acne, eczema and scars. It has an uplifting effect for depression and anxiety, and can help alleviate fluid retention.

Uses Inhalation, baths and massage. Small quantities will have a stimulating effect; larger doses sedate. Often worn as a perfume and used for an exotic, sensual massage.

PEPPERMINT
Mentha piperata

Origins The Egyptians used this aromatic herb in flavouring wine and food and valued its menthol content. Culpeper recorded in the seventeenth century that it was the herb most useful for "complaints of the stomach, such as wind and vomiting, for which there are few remedies of greater efficacy".

Description The leaves of peppermint are shorter and broader than spearmint with larger spikes of purple flowers. A British classic, it has spread throughout the world. The almost colourless peppermint oil is distilled from the whole of the partially dried plant and has a strong refreshing fragrance.

Therapeutic effects Excellent for the digestion, as a decongestant, and for skin disorders. Use for colds, flu, flatulence, headaches, indigestion, nausea, toothache and sunburn.

Uses Inhalation, baths and massage. Peppermint oil is still used in gripe water to settle upset stomachs. A few drops on a handkerchief can alleviate headaches and symptoms of sea and travel sickness, as it is refreshing and invigorating. It makes a refreshing skin tonic or bath oil in the summer because of its cooling properties. Used in a footbath it can help sweaty, smelly or tired feet, or in a compress to relieve hot flushes.

Cautionary note For skin complaints do not use in a concentration of more than one per cent as it can cause irritation.

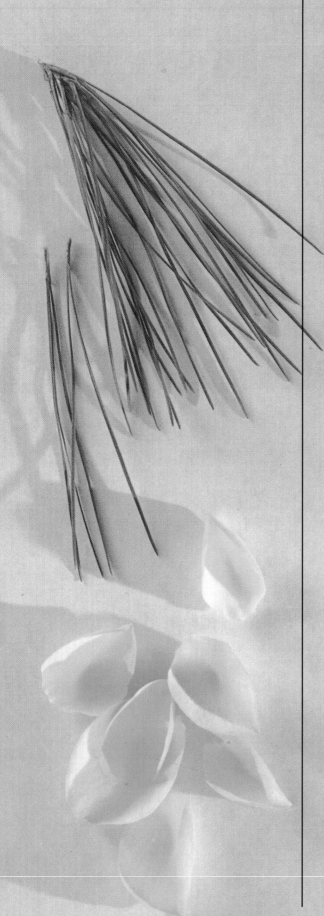

PINE
Pinus sylvestris

Origins The Scandinavians have traditionally used pine in the sauna or steam bath for its refreshing and antiseptic qualities.

Description This species of conifer grows wild all over Europe, North America and the USSR. General pine oil comes from the heart of the wood but the best essences are distilled from the pine needle. The oil has a fresh fragrance with a resinous woody undertone.

Therapeutic effects Acts as an antiseptic, and is particularly valuable for treating the respiratory tract, for bronchitis, catarrh, colds and sinusitis. Will also help relieve cystitis, arthritis and muscular aches and pains.

Uses Inhalation, baths and massage. Widely used to give coniferous fragrance in household products and in some masculine perfumes, this oil is popularly used throughout the cosmetics and pharmaceutical industries in balms, body rubs, soaps and bath oils. The oil can be used as an antiseptic deodorizer (add a few drops to freshen shoes) and in saunas or hot tubs for its invigorating steam.

ROSE
Rosa centifolia, Rosa damascena

Origins The rose has been loved for its fragrance at least since Roman times, when it was used in garlands, scented baths and perfumes, often in ostentatious public displays. But the rose has its private uses too: Cleopatra reputedly carpeted her bedroom in rose petals to aid her seduction of Mark Antony.

Description The Damascena rose is cultivated in Bulgaria. The flowers are picked at dawn and the yellowy-brown oil is extracted within 24 hours. It takes approximately five tons (five tonnes) of blossoms to produce just 2 lb (1 kg) of oil – not surprisingly one of the most expensive in the world. Centifolia roses, also yielding a richly fragrant oil, are cultivated in France, Algeria, Morocco and Eygpt.

Therapeutic effects An aphrodisiac and mood enhancer, rose is a general tonic and fortifier, useful for circulatory problems, constipation, headaches and mental fatigue, menstrual and menopausal problems and skin disorders.

Uses Baths and massage. One of the least toxic of all essences, it is particularly good for older, drier, skins, and is useful for pot pourri or to perfume bed linens and underwear (add a few drops to the final rinse).

ROSEMARY
Rosmarinus officinalis

Origins First favoured by the Egyptians, rosemary was popular with the Greeks and Romans who believed it symbolized love and death. During the plague it was burned in public places and worn around the neck for its antiseptic qualities.

Description A small shrub, it grows to around three feet (90 cm) high, with grey–green leaves and pale blue–white flowers. The clear oil is steam-distilled from the flowers and leaves, and has a powerful, warm, woody aroma.

Therapeutic effects A good stimulant, especially for the circulation and memory. Also helps alopecia, bronchitis, burns, colds, dandruff, diarrhoea, flatulence, headaches and obesity.

Uses Inhalation, baths and massage. Inhale from a handkerchief to clear headaches and fatigue. In massage it stimulates the lymphatic system.

Cautionary note Use in low concentration, as excessive doses may bring about epileptic fits or convulsions. Do not use in early pregnancy or if you have high blood pressure.

SAGE
Salvia officinalis, *Salvia sclarea* (Clary sage)

Origins A sacred herb, its properties were used by the Egyptians to help cure infertility in women. The Chinese have used it medicinally for centuries.

Description The many varieties of common sage are all shrub-like herbs with rough, wrinkled leaves. The oil is distilled from the dried leaves and has a powerful, fresh, spicy fragrance with a hint of camphor.

Therapeutic effects A tonic, particularly renowned for regulating menstruation, it can also help relieve arthritis, bacterial infections, throat infections and water retention.

Clary sage (*Salvia sclarea*) is also used for its sedative and euphoric effects, and in treating insomnia, anxiety and depression, as well as menstrual and menopausal problems. It has a spicy fragrance, rather more floral than common sage.

Uses Bathing and massage. A sage bath helps muscular aches and the effects of prolonged stress or mental strain.

Cautionary note In high doses, sage can overstimulate and should be avoided by anyone who suffers from epilepsy. Both sage and clary sage should be avoided in early pregnancy.

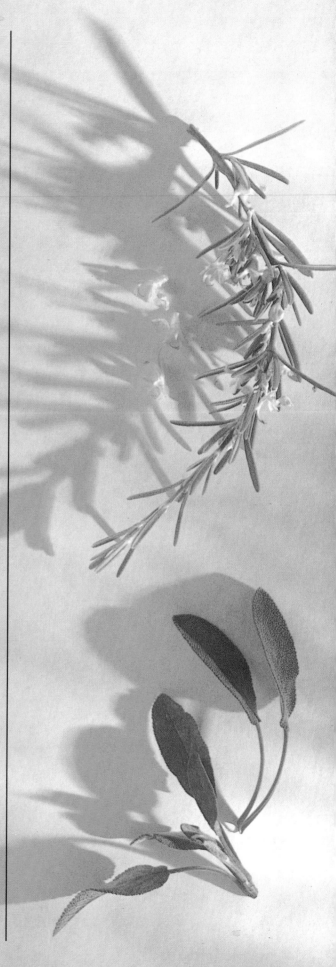

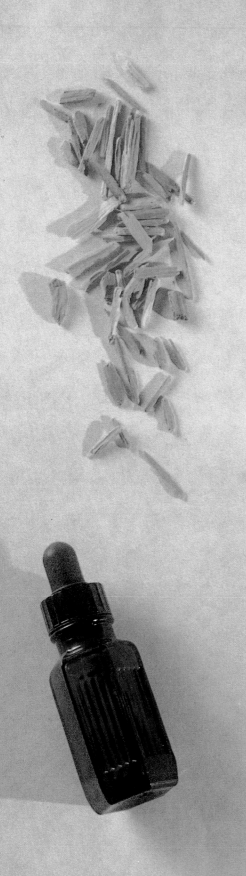

SANDALWOOD
Santalum album

Origins In China, India and Egypt sandalwood was used in perfumes and cosmetics. It has also been prized by furniture makers, and in India many of the temples were built with this lovely wood. Worshippers also covered their bodies with its essence, along with rose, jasmine and narcissus.

Description The evergreen sandalwood tree grows to a height of up to 30 feet (8 metres) in Indonesia, South East Asia and in particular East India. The syrupy, balsamic oil is extracted from the roughly chipped and powdered wood by steam distillation. It has a rich, warm, woody odour. It is used as a fixative in perfumes and gives the lingering classic base notes in many expensive fragrances.

Therapeutic effects Sandalwood's sedative properties are good for treating depression and tension. It is also an expectorant and anti-spasmodic; useful for bronchitis, coughs, nausea, cystitis and skin complaints. Regarded as an aphrodisiac.

Uses Inhalation and massage. Apply in a warm compress to revitalize dehydrated skin. Blends well with neroli and rose. Massage enhances its soothing effects.

TEA TREE
Melaleuca alternifolia

Origins The antiseptic properties of the tea tree were discovered centuries ago by the Aborigines of Australia who used it medicinally for treating sunburn and many bacterial/fungus infections, from ringworm to athlete's foot. It was known as an antidote for venomous snake bites.

Description A native of Australia and Tasmania, it is often referred to as the swamp tree. It produces white hanging flowers on a long spike, but the pale green oil is extracted from the twigs and leaves, which have a strong aromatic odour. The oil itself has a camphorous smell, reminiscent of eucalyptus.

Therapeutic effects A strong disinfectant and antiseptic, it is ideal for skin complaints including athlete's foot, burns, cold sores, mouth ulcers, verrucas, thrush and warts. Also effective for many respiratory complaints.

Uses Inhalation and baths. It can be used to kill fleas on pets but is more commonly used as a deodorizing/antiseptic foot bath. Dab on cold sores. Inhale to alleviate laryngitis and bronchitis. Diluted in water, it can be used as a mouthwash (not swallowed) to soothe ulcers.

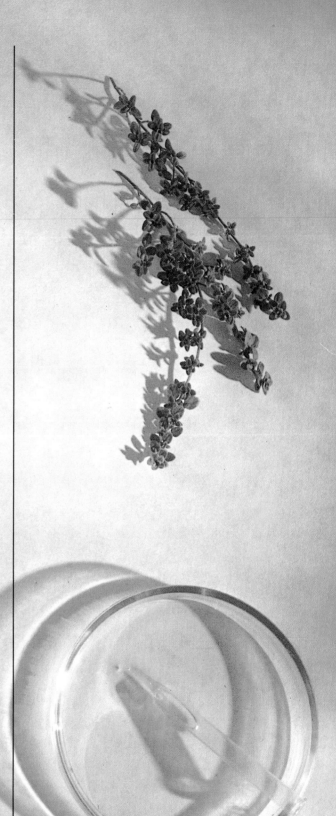

THYME
Thymus vulgaris

Origins The ancient Egyptians incorporated the essential oil of thyme into their embalming fluids. The Greeks drank a herbal infusion of the leaves after banquets to aid digestion. Culpeper considered it a great lung strengthener and a remedy for shortness of breath.

Description This common low-growing wild herb has dark green leaves, woody stalks and small pink flowers. It is cultivated throughout the Mediterranean, Algeria, Yugoslavia and in Egypt for culinary and pharmaceutical uses. The oil is extracted from the whole flowering herb by steam-distillation and has a pungent, sweet herbaceous smell. It is an important component in colognes and herbal perfumes.

Therapeutic effects Helps fatigue and anxiety, but best known as a natural antiseptic for treating coughs and infections of the respiratory tract. Good too for rheumatic aches and for skin problems such as sores and swellings.

Uses Massage and baths. When added to a bath, its invigorating effects help revive tired muscles.

YLANG-YLANG
Cananga odorata

Origins A tropical tree, its first medicinal uses were to treat malaria, soothe insect bites and generally fight infections. Its antiseptic qualities were appreciated but it was also recognized as an aphrodisiac and a tonic to the nervous system. In the past, the flowers were mixed with coconut oil to perfume and condition the body and hair.

Description A native of Indonesia and the Philippines, the ylang-ylang tree reaches a height of 60 feet (10 metres). The yellow flowers are freshly picked in the early morning and the oil extracted by steam-distillation. It has a narcotic, floral-sweet, jasmine-like aroma which adds warmth to perfumes.

Therapeutic effects A great relaxer (if used sparingly) and highly recommended for anxiety, depression, insomnia and frigidity. It also has benefits in treating high blood pressure and skin conditions.

Uses Baths and massage. This oil can soothe away all forms of stress when used as a bath oil or massaged onto the body. Its lasting fragrance is often used in facial and skin preparations, pot pourri and pomanders. It blends well with bergamot, melissa, sandalwood and jasmine.

33

OILS FOR COMMON PROBLEMS

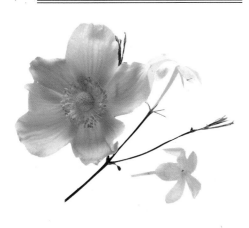

Oil	Type	Acne	Anxiety	Arthritis	Athlete's Foot	Blood pressure: High	Low	Body odour	Bronchitis	Cellulite	Colds/chills
Basil	R, U		❀						❀		❀
Bay	R			❀				❀	❀		
Benzoin	S			❀				❀	❀		❀
Bergamot	R, U	❀	❀								
Cedarwood	R	❀							❀		
Chamomile	R	❀	❀	❀							
Cinnamon	R							❀			❀
Comfrey	R				❀						
Cypress	R		❀					❀		❀	
Eucalyptus	S	❀		❀				❀			❀
Fennel	S										
Frankincense	R										❀
Geranium	R, U		❀								❀
Hyssop	R, S					❀	❀		❀		❀
Jasmine	R		❀								
Juniper	R, U	❀	❀							❀	
Lavender	R, U	❀	❀	❀	❀	❀		❀	❀		❀
Lemon	S	❀					❀				❀
Lemongrass	S	❀			❀			❀			
Marjoram	R		❀	❀		❀			❀		
Melissa	R, U		❀			❀					
Myrrh	S								❀		❀
Neroli	R		❀					❀			
Orange	U		❀			❀					
Parsley	S										
Patchouli	R	❀	❀		❀					❀	
Peppermint	S						❀	❀	❀		
Pine	S			❀					❀	❀	❀
Rose	R		❀	❀							
Rosemary	S						❀			❀	❀
Sage	S		❀	❀			❀		❀		
Clary Sage	R, S		❀			❀					
Sandalwood	R	❀	❀						❀		
Tea Tree	S				❀				❀		❀
Thyme	S		❀						❀		
Ylang-Ylang	R		❀			❀					

Water retention									❀				❀			❀	❀								❀			❀		❀	❀					
Warts																	❀	❀									❀							❀		
Varicose veins									❀							❀		❀	❀								❀			❀						
Travel sickness																	❀																			
Throat infections				❀						❀		❀	❀				❀	❀	❀			❀									❀	❀	❀	❀		
Stress						❀							❀				❀			❀	❀						❀						❀			
Sinusitus										❀							❀						❀					❀								
Sexual problems					❀		❀						❀		❀											❀			❀			❀	❀			❀
Rheumatism		❀				❀			❀	❀						❀	❀	❀		❀			❀					❀		❀					❀	
Pre-menstrual syndrome	❀					❀			❀				❀			❀	❀				❀		❀						❀	❀	❀	❀	❀		❀	
Obesity									❀		❀															❀				❀	❀				❀	
Nausea	❀										❀						❀				❀						❀		❀				❀			
Muscular aches							❀	❀	❀	❀							❀			❀								❀		❀	❀					
Mental fatigue	❀															❀					❀							❀		❀	❀	❀			❀	
Painful periods						❀		❀	❀						❀	❀				❀	❀								❀			❀				
Irregular periods						❀										❀	❀				❀								❀	❀	❀	❀				
Menstrual problems (general)	❀					❀								❀		❀	❀				❀								❀	❀		❀			❀	
Menopausal problems						❀		❀	❀		❀		❀				❀	❀			❀		❀	❀					❀		❀	❀				
Insomnia					❀	❀			❀			❀		❀			❀			❀			❀						❀			❀	❀			
Influenza	❀						❀		❀	❀				❀														❀						❀		
Indigestion	❀					❀										❀	❀	❀	❀	❀	❀	❀		❀			❀			❀						
Hormonal regulation						❀							❀								❀			❀												
Headache	❀					❀				❀							❀		❀	❀	❀						❀			❀						
Hayfever						❀				❀											❀								❀							
Haemorrhoids									❀													❀					❀						❀			
Flatulence				❀		❀					❀			❀		❀	❀	❀									❀			❀		❀			❀	
Fainting	❀					❀											❀										❀			❀						
Eczema					❀	❀		❀	❀				❀	❀	❀	❀						❀				❀							❀			
Diarrhoea						❀	❀		❀	❀			❀			❀	❀	❀			❀	❀					❀									
Depression	❀			❀		❀			❀				❀		❀		❀		❀				❀	❀		❀			❀	❀	❀	❀	❀			❀
Dandruff					❀								❀			❀	❀	❀								❀				❀			❀	❀		
Cystitis			❀	❀					❀	❀						❀									❀			❀			❀		❀			
Constipation						❀					❀									❀				❀					❀	❀						

THE ESSENTIAL MASSAGE

An aromatherapy massage using essential oils is a therapeutic treatment for both mind and body which works mainly on the nervous system. Aromatherapy is both holistic and practical in that it helps to protect the body's life-saving immune system and energize or stabilize emotions. It is often called the "sensual science" because it combines the powers of touch with the sense of smell. More effectively than any other massage, aromatherapy can either relax or stimulate the body and mind. The highly potent essential oils penetrate the body via the skin and are also inhaled as the massage progresses.

SETTING UP

Any massage is relaxing but you can enhance the experience by following a few simple steps to help create the right mood.

An aromatherapist uses a massage bench, but at home you can work comfortably on a cushioned floor or a futon (Japanese mattress). An ordinary bed is not really firm enough. Prepare the floor or surface with a large cotton sheet covered with a bath towel. You should also have to hand a pillow, a large wrap-around towel for the body, and a warm blanket or even a hot-water bottle by the feet.

RELAXING YOUR PARTNER

Additional touches help to establish a calming atmosphere. You could fragrance the room with a burner, using a relaxing oil, and switch on some background music: play instrumental tracks, as voices can distract any train of thought.

The room temperature should be warm. Once the oils are gently massaged in, the whole body responds by slowing down and, although the skin may feel warm to touch, the body feels colder. It is important to keep your partner comfortable, so offer to cover parts that are not being worked on if you think your partner may be getting cold. Being at ease with one another is an important part of any treatment.

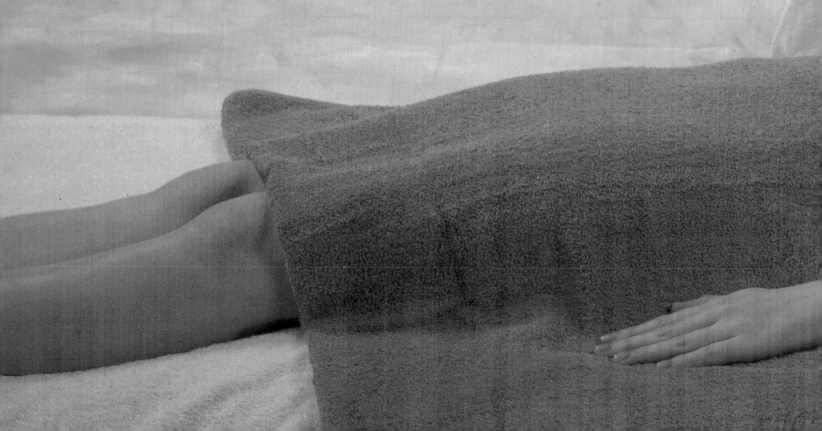

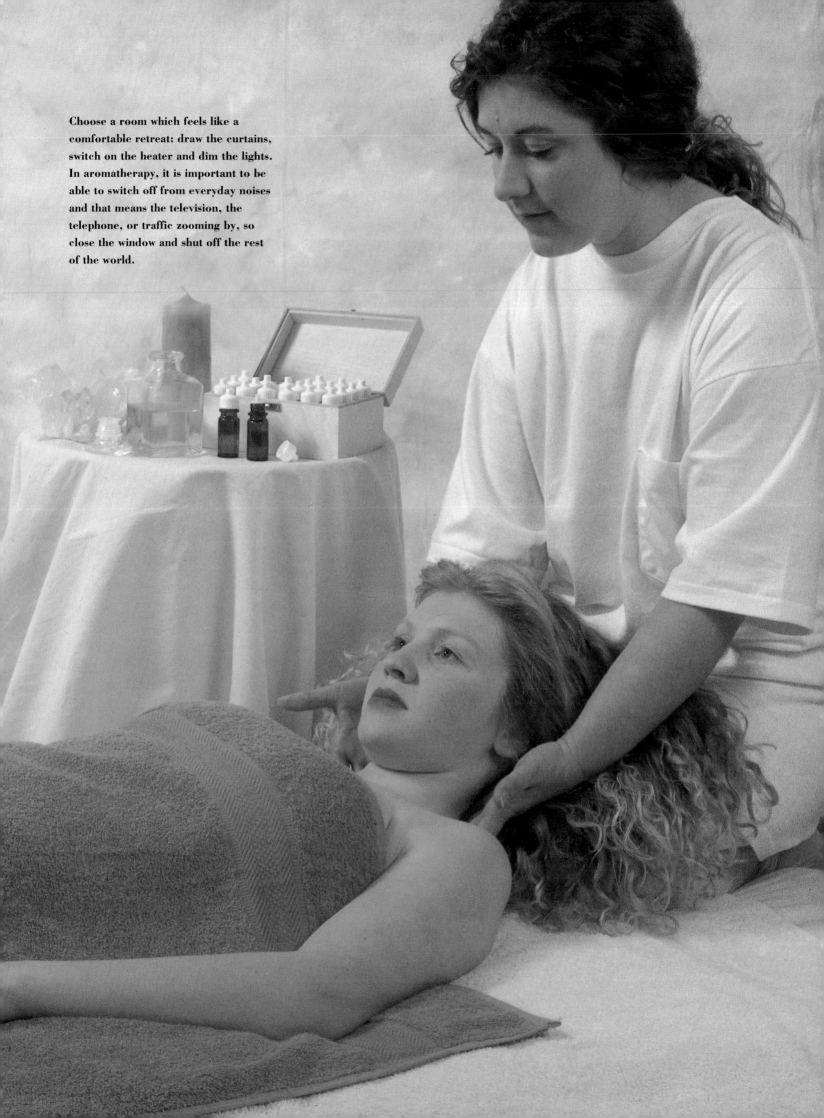

Choose a room which feels like a comfortable retreat: draw the curtains, switch on the heater and dim the lights. In aromatherapy, it is important to be able to switch off from everyday noises and that means the television, the telephone, or traffic zooming by, so close the window and shut off the rest of the world.

ABOUT THE TREATMENT

A complete aromatherapy massage takes just under an hour from top to toe. It is important to find out before massage about physical aches and pains, in particular back injuries, recent operations or whether the person you are massaging is in an "emotional" state of mind at the time.

GIVING THE MASSAGE

● Make sure you have read through the step-by-step instructions several times to familiarize yourself with the sequence. You don't want to keep stopping to refer to the book.

● Try out the movements on parts of your own body to get a sense of how the strokes should feel and how much pressure to use.

● Massage movements should be slow and gentle to help relaxation and eliminate tension which tightens the muscles.

● Remember that the movements should flow into each other. If you find you have missed out a step or gone on to the wrong part of the body, don't panic. Finish the part you are working on before going back to it, or leave it out altogether, rather than interrupting the flow of the massage.

● When you give the massage, make sure *you* are relaxed and comfortable, as well as the person you're working on, or you will transmit your own tensions to your partner and it will not be an effective massage.

● Try to maintain contact with your partner's body as much as possible; even as you move into a different position try to keep a hand on the body.

● When massaging different parts of the body keep the areas not being worked on covered with a large towel or blanket. The heat helps the body to absorb the oils.

CHOOSING THE ESSENTIAL OIL

romatherapists never start a massage immediately. In order to provide the most effective treatment, the therapist has to ascertain the state of mind and body of the individual, and establish whether there are any specific problems to attend to. Is the problem physical? Is it mental? Is it a combination of both? To help them to treat a wide variety of complaints, aromatherapists have many oils at their fingertips, but they never mix or use them until they have worked out a prescription for the receiver's individual needs.

Mixing the oils is a trained art, yet there are simple recipes you can use at home to deal with specific problems from muscular aches and pains to headaches and stress. With potent essential oils it is far better to use less, rather than more, so if in doubt, start the massage technique with a base oil like sweet almond and add two or three drops of just one essential oil. Lavender, rosemary and geranium are good all-purpose oils, or use chamomile for particularly sensitive skin.

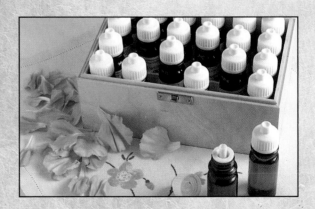

APPLYING THE OILS

 eep the oil in an easy dispenser or bowl so you don't have to worry about lids during the massage. But keep the oil covered in some way as essential oils will quickly evaporate.

● Always warm your hands before applying oils.

● Some therapists recommend warming the oil in your hands before applying it to the body as a courtesy to the recipient. Others advise against this on the grounds that it hastens evaporation of the essential oil and that the oil takes on your own energy rather than your partner's.

● If the part of the body you're working on is particularly hairy or the skin is very dry you will need to apply more oil.

● Keep your touch light and sensitive. Remember that your hands are the main channel of communication.

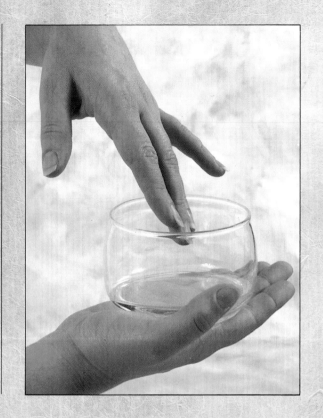

● If the recipient's back is stressed in any way, place a pillow under the knees when lying on the back, and under the pelvis when lying on the stomach.

● Wear loose comfortable clothing to give the massage, so your movements are not hampered.

● If oil is accidentally spilt on clothing, dab off quickly with a tissue. It will soon evaporate, but it may leave a stain so rinse out clothing in warm soapy water.

● For complete relaxation avoid chatting during the massage: play music if you don't like silence. But do encourage feedback from your partner – you must be told if something doesn't feel good.

● Ensure that the person you are going to work on is given the following set of guidelines.

RECEIVING THE MASSAGE

Before the Massage

● Have a cool shower or wash before a massage. Do not soak in a hot bath, or the oils will immediately seep into the skin.

● Don't use an underarm deodorant or body spray during the treatment, as this will block the effect of the oils.

● Don't have a large meal just before an aromatherapy massage as the body's systems will have to work too hard at digesting to be thoroughly relaxed.

● Don't drink alcohol before a treatment.

● Don't have a massage if you have flu or a fever or any serious condition (*see* Cautions). Wait until you are over the worst and

then let an aromatherapy treatment help restore your system's balance.

After the Massage

● Drink a glass of still water immediately after a treatment.

● Lie still for at least five minutes before getting up.

● Don't bathe or shower for at least twelve hours after a treatment to allow the oils to be absorbed by the skin and begin the all-important work of detoxifying the body.

● Drink plenty of water for the rest of the day as the kidneys will be active in eliminating the toxins.

● Avoid alcohol for at least 12 hours after the treatment to give the body a chance to detoxify thoroughly.

THE MASSAGE STEP-BY-STEP

Following your assessment, select the oils you are going to use and blend 10–15 drops of your chosen oils with four tablespoons of base oil.

The massage starts with your partner lying face down, with the back uncovered and the rest of the body covered with a towel or light blanket.

ESTABLISHING CONTACT

Take a few moments to create a bond of communication with your partner and to prepare yourself for the massage. Focus or "centre" yourself by becoming aware of your whole body and its role in giving the massage, and letting go of outside concerns to concentrate on the task in hand.

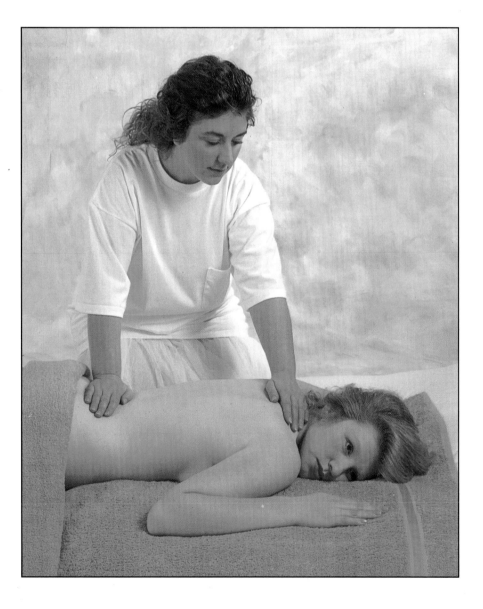

═══ CAUTIONS ═══

Aromatherapy is an holistic therapy in that it works on the person as a whole. Though it is an excellent way of treating minor ailments, stress and negative emotional states, it is not a substitute for conventional medical treatment. If symptoms persist, always consult a medical doctor.

Never attempt to treat the following conditions:
- cancer
- progressive neural disorders
- heart conditions
- advanced asthmatic conditions
- post-operative states
- severe varicose veins
- very high blood pressure
- epilepsy

For oils to avoid during pregnancy *see* Pregnancy Treatments.

Left: With your partner face down, rest one hand lightly at the base of the neck (the occipital bone) and place your other hand on the lower back (the sacral area). Hold the position for a count of 20, while you focus on your breathing and clear your mind. This is carried out with dry hands.

THE LEG

EFFLEURAGE (SMOOTHING STROKE)

This is a smooth, sliding movement which soothes the skin and distributes the oil. Always worked in the direction of the heart, effleurage improves circulation, lymph flow and the function of the muscles. It is used between movements throughout the massage to provide continuity and to prepare a new area with oil.

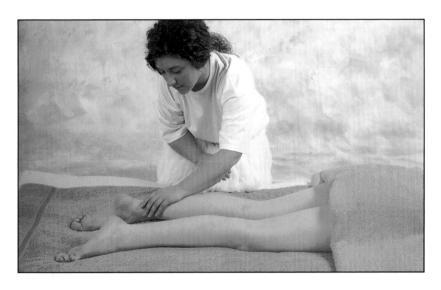

1 *Seated to the side of your partner, begin with one hand at the heel, brushing in an* upward, sweeping movement to the buttock ridge and sliding round to the thigh.

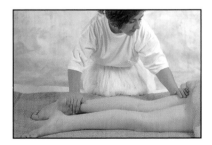 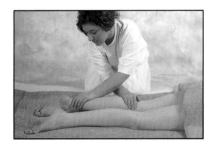

2 *As the first hand comes round the thigh, place the other hand at the heel and brush with an upward sweep, ending at the back of the knee.*

3 *As the second hand comes off, cross the first hand over and begin the movement again from the heel up to the thigh.*

Repeat the sequence about six or seven times, keeping the movements continuous and flowing, and then repeat on the other leg.

ANKLE THUMBING

The ankles are an important centre of energy, and this movement helps to relieve congestion.

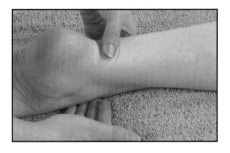

1 *Sitting at your partner's feet, cradle one ankle gently with your hands, allowing the thumbs to sit naturally above the heel.*

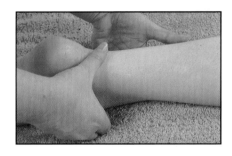

2 *Keeping the rest of the hand still, apply a light pressure with the thumb as it brushes in an upward and outward movement.*

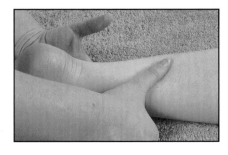

3 *Repeat with alternate thumbs, continuing in a rhythmic sequence for about 30 seconds.*

FLUSHING

Flushing drains the lymph channels and stimulates the circulation.
This movement should not be used on anyone with severe varicose veins.

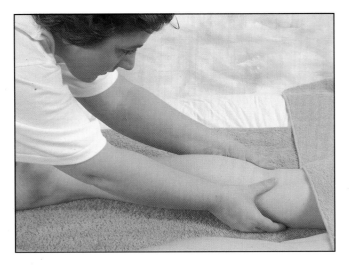

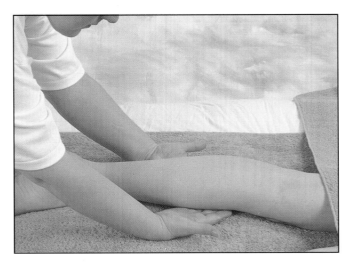

1 *Sitting at your partner's feet, gently slide the thumbs up the middle of the leg, ending at the back of the knee.*

2 *Slowly bring the hands back down to the ankles by brushing down the sides of the calf muscle, taking care not to drag.*

Repeat the movement five or six times.

KNEADING

Move back round to the side of the leg for this movement. It is particularly effective for relieving tension at the back of the legs.

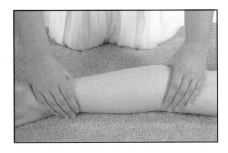

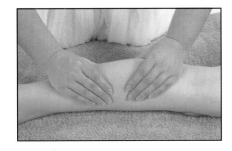

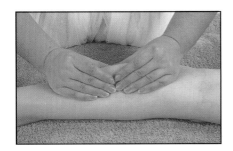

1 *Place the hands gently on the calf, one at the top and one just above the ankle.*

2 *Grasp the calf muscle firmly with both hands and slide them toward the centre of the calf, lifting the muscle.*

3 *Using gentle pressure, knead the area by bringing the fingers and thumbs together and raising the muscle further.*

Continue kneading for about 30 seconds.

WRINGING

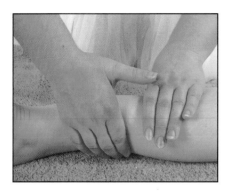

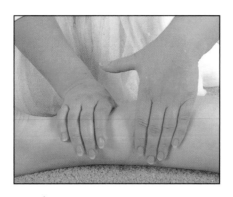

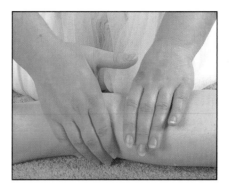

1 *Place the hands on opposite sides of the calf, just above the ankle. Gently glide the hands past each other so the heel of one hand is pushing away from you while the other hand is pulling.*

2 *Keep the thumb of the pulling hand raised so the thumbs don't collide as they pass each other each time.*

3 *The hands alternate the pushing and pulling as you work all the way up the calf and down again. The pressure should be firm but gentle.*

Clear these movements by flushing through again from ankle to back of knee.

THUMBING THE KNEE

This is the same action as the thumbing performed at the ankle base. It is helpful for people who suffer from cold feet as it stimulates the circulation.

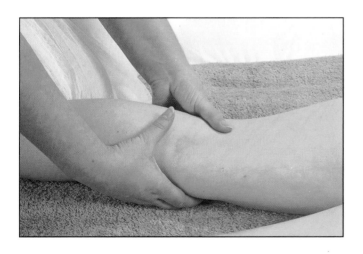

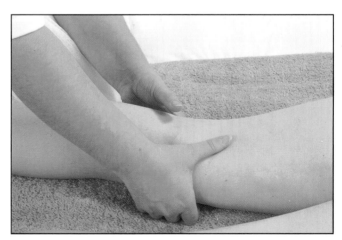

1 *Cup the hands gently around the knee, allowing the thumbs to sit naturally on the fleshy part at the back of the knee.*

2 *With the same thumbing movement used on the ankles, brush one thumb upward and outward, covering the full width of the knee, and follow immediately with the opposite thumb.*

FLUSHING

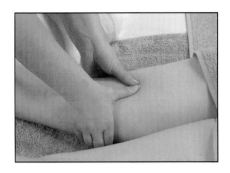

Flush through with the thumbs together from the back of the knee to the top of the thigh.

WRINGING

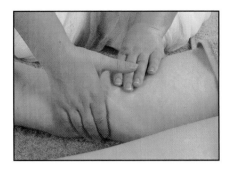

Wring the leg from the knee to the top of the thigh with the same action as used on the lower leg.

THIGH PUSH

This knuckling movement is very effective for breaking down cellulite, helping to disperse the fatty tissue and improve the circulation.

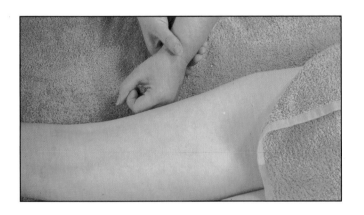

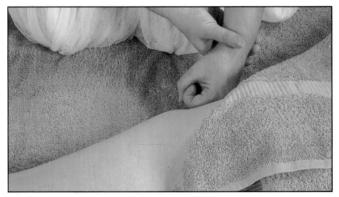

1 *With the supporting hand wrapped around the wrist of the working hand for stability, place the clenched fist on the side of the thigh, just above the knee.*

2 *Drag the fist slowly up the side of the thigh toward the hip bone. This is not a heavy action – all you need is gentle pressure.*

Repeat five or six times, working slightly different parts of the thigh each time.

Finish the leg massage by repeating the opening effluerage movement and then repeat all the steps on the other leg.

Cover the legs with towels before proceeding to the next stage. An extra blanket or hot water bottle at the feet might also be appreciated.

BACK MASSAGE

The back carries a lot of strain and these relaxing movements are often the most appreciated part of the massage. Don't be tempted to use too much pressure: it is better to keep the strokes broad and flowing.

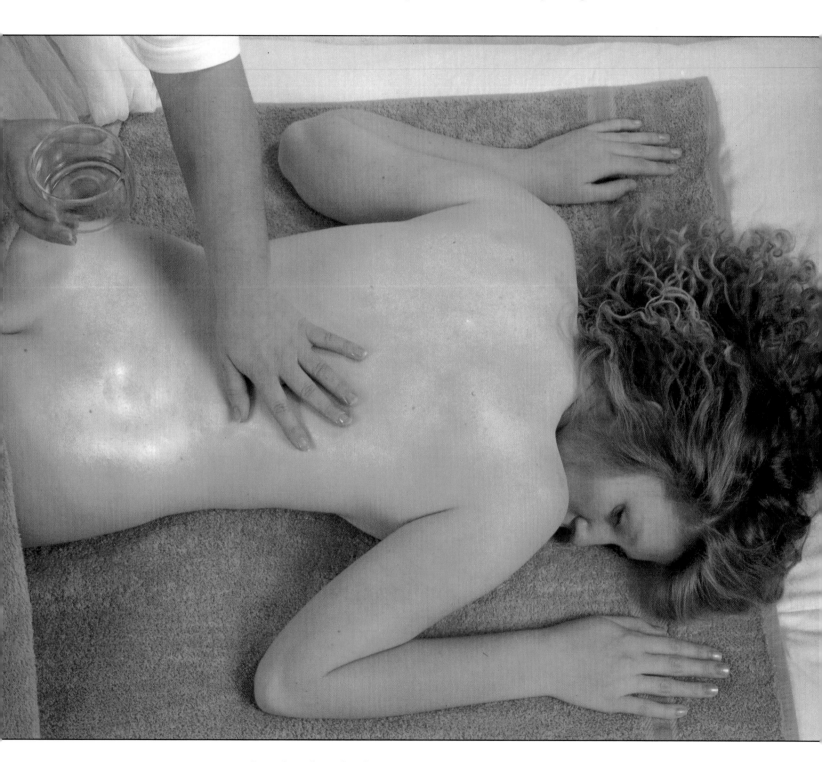

Seated to the side of your partner, apply oil evenly over the back with smooth upward strokes, following the direction of the lymph flow.

FIGURE-OF-EIGHT

This sequence loosens the tissue all over the back and helps to stimulate
blood and lymph flow, and relieve tension.

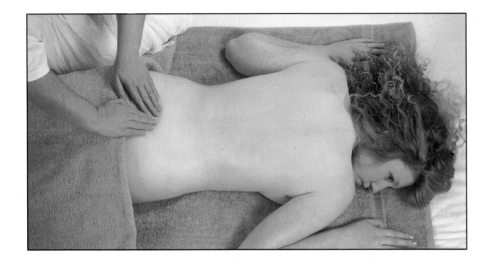

You should be kneeling level with
the buttocks, facing the head so
that you can lean into the
movement and reach the shoulders
without straining.

1 To begin this large sweeping
movement, place both hands on
the lower back, just above the base
of the spine, fingers pointing
toward the head.

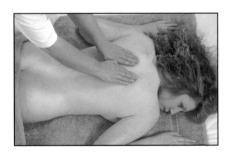

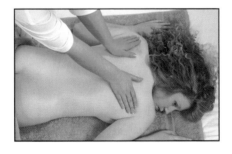

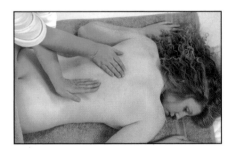

2 Slide both hands all the way
up the sides of the spine to just
below the base of the neck.

3 Move the hands out around
the shoulders and in toward
each other across the upper back.

4 As the hands pass each other,
cross the right arm over the left
and continue gliding.

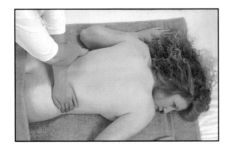

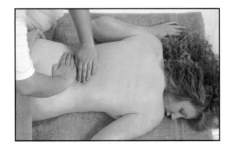

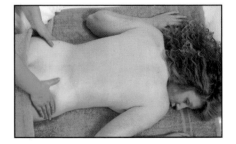

5 With arms still crossed, reach
down around the waist.

6 Pull the flesh-up firmly
around the waist and then
gradually release the sides as the
palms glide to the middle of the
lower back and pass each other.

7 Continue the movement by
sliding the palms out around
the hips and complete the figure-of-
eight by returning the hands to the
starting position.

Repeat six times, always keeping the movements broad and flowing.

FANNING

This action works on the nerves along the spine and helps to disperse the fluid that accumulates in the back tissue as a result of tension. The effect is wonderfully relaxing.

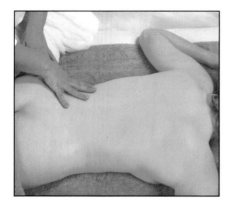

1 *Place one hand on the lower back, at the base of the spine. The fingers should be splayed open, with the index finger pointing to the side of the spine.*

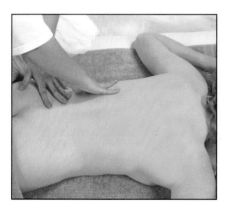

2 *Fan the hand round in an upward and outward motion away from the spine. The other hand follows on the same side as the first completes the movement. Work all the way up the side of the spine, alternating hands.*

Repeat the steps four or five times before moving round to work on the other side of the spine.

BUTTERFLY SHOULDERS

Before being given an aromatherapy massage, always wash off any anti-perspirant or deodorant. This is particularly important for this movement as it drains the lymph towards the major lymph glands in the armpits – the axillary glands. This movement relaxes the shoulder and disperses tension.

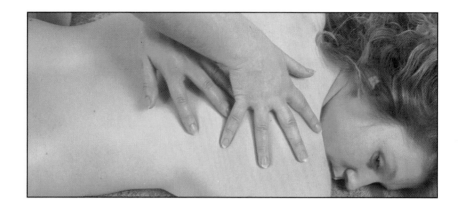

1 *Place one hand at the bottom of the shoulder blade (scapula) with fingers splayed and the second hand poised to follow on the same side.*

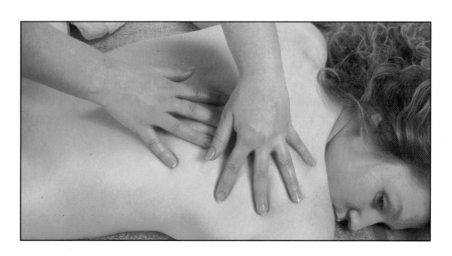

2 *Brush the hand up and out in a smooth fanning movement. Follow with the second hand, work all round the shoulder blade and out over the shoulder, toward the armpit.*

Repeat the whole movement four times, then work on the other shoulder.

FOREARM SWEEP

Kneeling at the side of your partner, turn the head away from you.

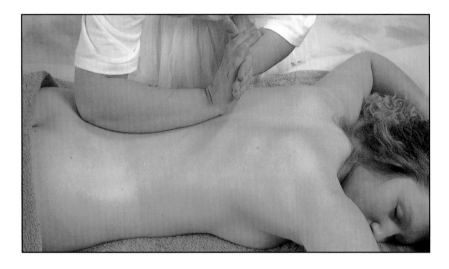

1 *Place your forearm alongside the spine with your elbow just above the buttocks. Clasp the working hand with your other hand for support and stability.*

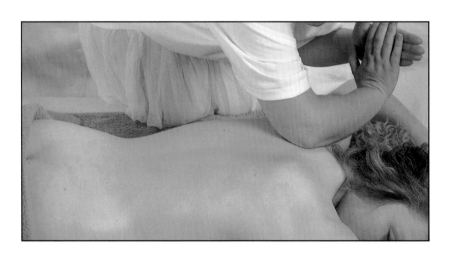

2 *Using the flat bone of the forearm (the ulna), slide all the way up the side of the spine to the top of the shoulder ridge.*

Lift the arm off gently and repeat twice from the beginning.

Then turn your partner's head and work on the other side of the spine, using the opposite forearm.

DRAINING

Sit to the side of your partner, facing across the back.

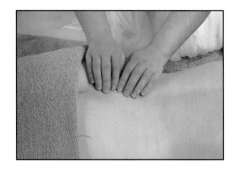

1 *With hands together and palms raised, place the fingertips at the side of the spine, just above the coccyx (tail bone).*

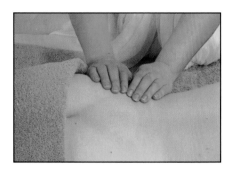

2 *Keeping the fingers together, pull them toward you down the side of the back.*

Repeat the movement all the way up the spine, ending at the base of the neck so the final movement pulls across the shoulders toward the glands in the armpit.

Repeat with the other side of the spine. You can work the opposite side without changing your position by reaching across and brushing away from the spine, or you can move around your partner and repeat as above, if it feels more comfortable.

KNEADING THE NECK

This gentle petrissage *movement releases tension and helps disperse the fatty deposits that can build up in this sensitive area.*

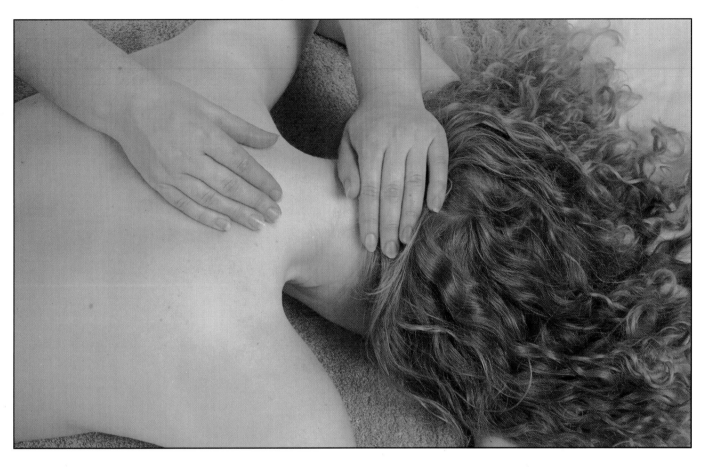

Your partner should rest facing down with forehead on hands, so that you can work your fingers into the base of the neck. Smooth the hair away from the neck.

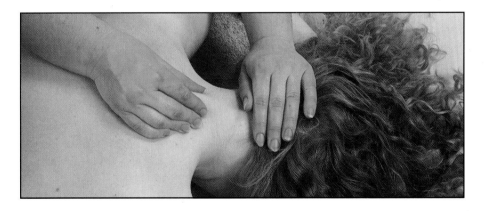

Resting one hand gently on the back of the head, use the other hand to pull up and knead the muscles in *the base of the neck (the occipitals), rolling the muscle between the thumb and the other fingers.*

49

FRONTAL MASSAGE

Help your partner to turn over onto their back, and ensure he or she is comfortable.
Provide cushions or rolled towels for any parts that need support,
such as behind the legs or neck. Cover the body up to the neck
with a towel or blanket to keep your partner warm.

SPINAL STRETCH

This movement is not suitable for people suffering from severe
back problems, though it helps relieve minor aches and stiffness.

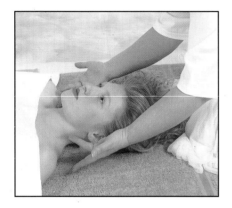

1 *Seated at your partner's head, place the hands to the sides of the neck, palms up, with the middle fingers lifted, to prepare for the movement.*

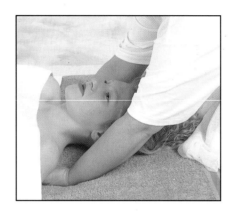

2 *Slide the hands underneath the back, just between the shoulder blades so the middle fingers are pressing on either side of the spine.*

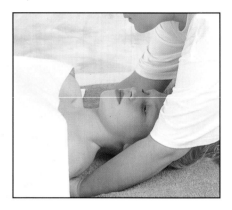

3 *Gently lift the torso so the rib cage rises, maintaining the pressure from the middle fingers.*

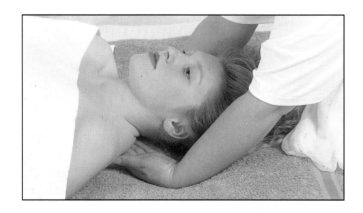

4 *Slowly pull your fingers up the sides of the spine. When you reach the top of the neck, hold for a count of two and then release. Repeat three times in all.*

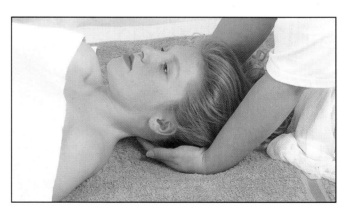

5 *Finish the movement by cradling the head gently with both hands.*

THE FACE

This treatment is a great boost to the circulation, and the complexion
will improve with each treatment.

Seated at the head, prepare the face for the massage with a simple refreshing cleanser, using upward and outward strokes. Apply a small amount of facial oil to the face and neck with flowing movements.

═══TAKE CARE═══

Even when diluted, essential oils are extremely potent so work carefully around the eye area. If the oil accidentally makes contact with the eye, apply a few drops of pure sweet almond oil to dissipate it. Never wash the eyes with water.

FOREHEAD STROKE

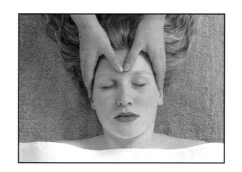
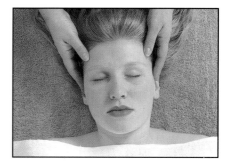

1 *Rest your thumbs on the centre of the forehead, just above the eyebrows, with the palms supporting the sides of the head. The stroke should be kept light and sensitive as the facial skin is very delicate.*

2 *Slowly draw the thumbs out toward the temples and down to the sides of the ears. Repeat the stroke several times, moving the starting position up a little each time until you reach the hairline.*

DRAINING THE CHEEKS

This sequence of raking movements stimulates the lymphatic flow in the face, improving the complexion, clearing the sinuses and releasing tension.

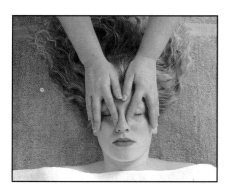
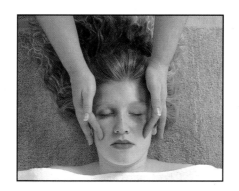
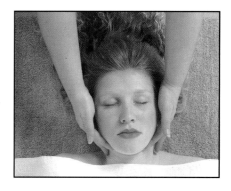

1 *Place the index fingers on either side of the nostrils and hold for a count of five.*

2 *Slide the fingers out and down to the ears. Lift the fingers and replace by the nostril. Sweep in a slightly narrower curve to reach the jawbone just below the ears.*

3 *Repeat with successively smaller curves, ending by tracing the laughter lines around the mouth, downward to the sides of the chin.*

CHIN MASSAGE

This not only tones the jawline, but also stimulates the energy points that govern the stomach and small intestine.

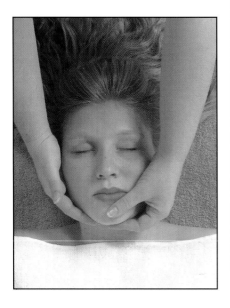

1 Place the thumbs on the chin, allowing the rest of the fingers to cradle the jaw.

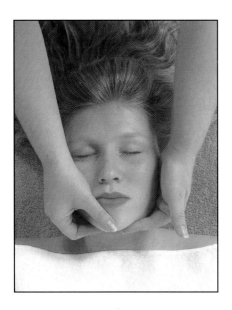

2 Brush alternate thumbs down and outward, with a light stroke. Repeat the movement six or seven times with each thumb.

NECK SWEEP

This is an extremely soothing stroke which improves the tone of the muscles as well as flushing the neck.

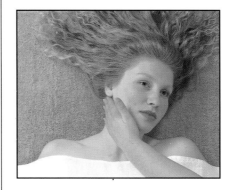

1,2 *Above and right:* Apply a little facial oil to the neck, upper chest and shoulder areas using the flat of the hand. Gently brush down with the hand from the side of the ear out to the shoulder, using a broad sweeping stroke to cover the area.

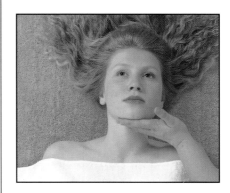

3 Repeat the movement working round the front of the neck, down from the chin to the top of the chest, and then sweep from the other ear to the shoulder.

The sequence of sweeps round the whole neck should be repeated three times.

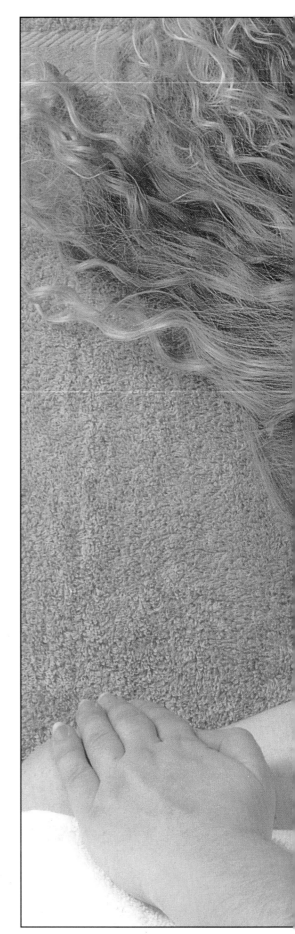

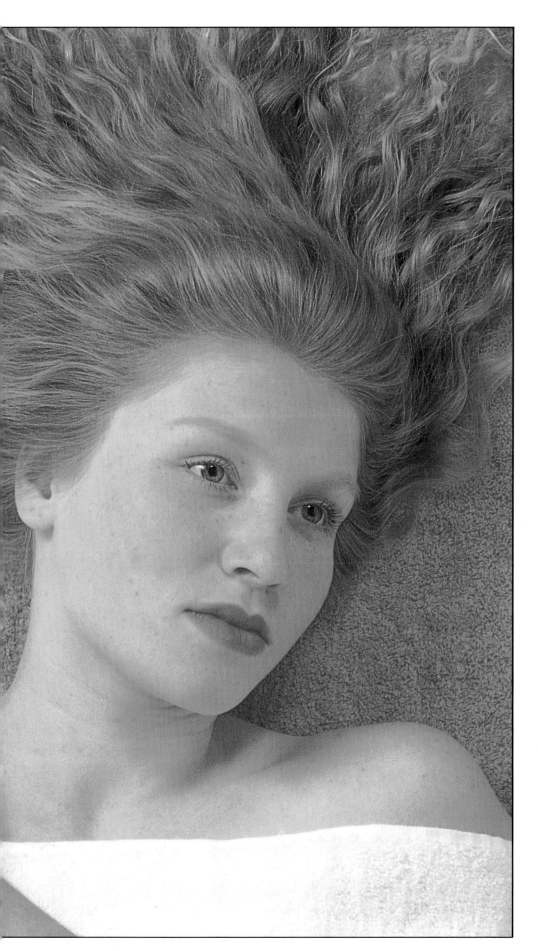

FANNING THE SHOULDERS

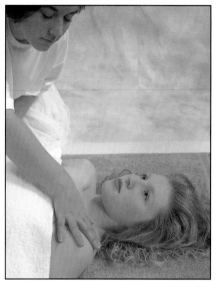

1 *With fingers spread, brush with the flat of the hand across from the breastbone and out over the shoulders.*

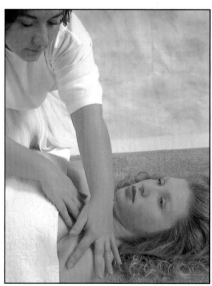

2 *The second hand follows closely behind the first, so they are draining simultaneously toward the armpit.*

Repeat twice before moving onto the other shoulder.

STOMACH AREA

ABDOMEN

1 *Left: Apply a little oil evenly over the stomach. Place the palm of a hand on the centre of the abdomen.*

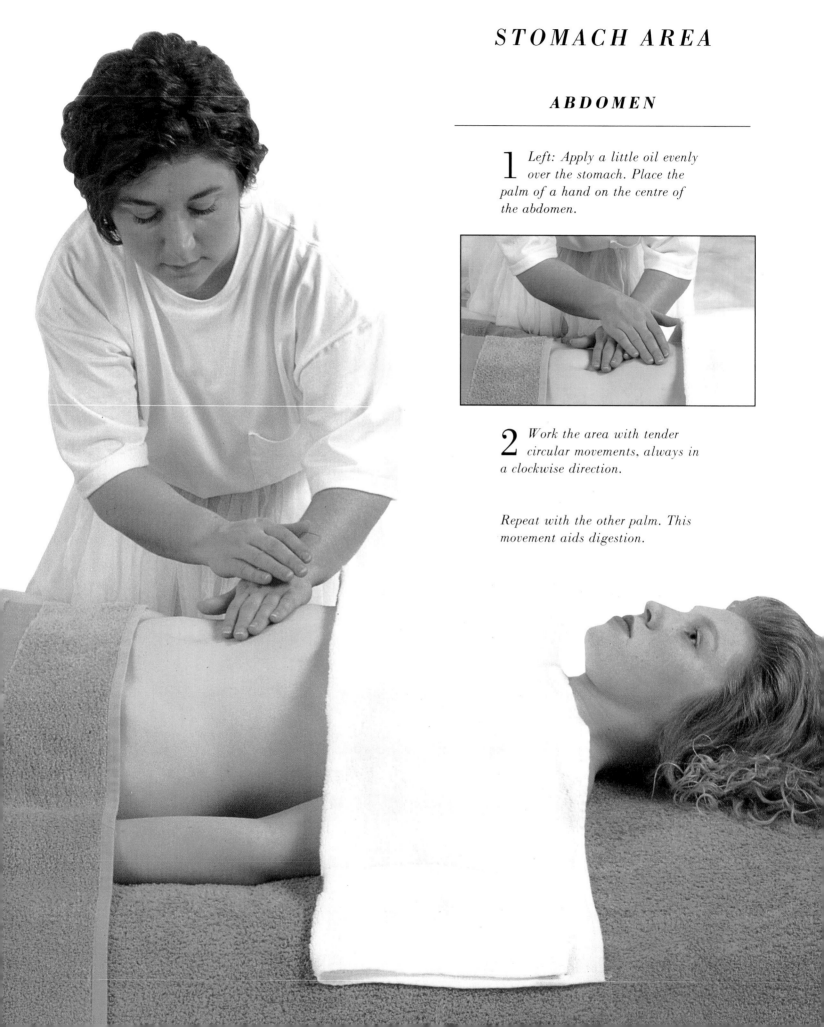

2 *Work the area with tender circular movements, always in a clockwise direction.*

Repeat with the other palm. This movement aids digestion.

RIB-CAGE SWEEP

This movement helps to cleanse the stomach and spleen by pushing the lymph away from these areas.

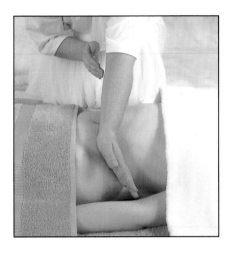

1 *Starting with the outer edge of the hand placed at the centre of the rib-cage, sweep away from you, following the line of the ribs with a long sweeping movement out to the waist.*

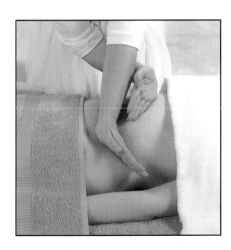

2 *As the first hand finishes the movement, the other hand follows on the same side.*

Repeat the movement with both hands six or seven times and then move around the body to work the other side of the rib-cage.

WAIST PULLS

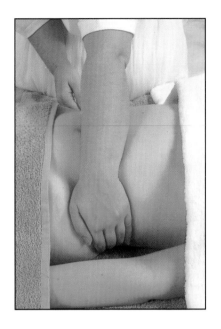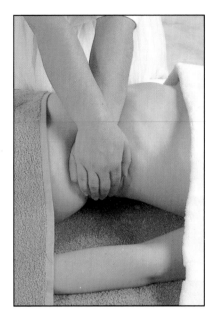

1 *Reach across your partner, placing a firm grip round the waist with one hand. Reinforce your grip by placing your other hand on top of the first hand.*

2 *Lift the waist by pulling your partner's body-weight toward you, then gently release while sliding the hands around the hipbone. This cleanses the liver and gall bladder.*

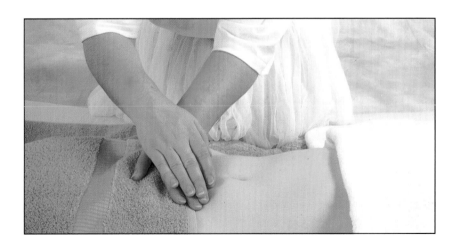

3 *Complete the movement by sliding the hands across and around the pelvis, draining toward the major glands in the groin. Be careful not to dig with the fingers as this is an* *extremely tender area. Keep the pressure light and even over the whole hand. This is particularly beneficial for women who suffer from menstrual problems.*

Repeat five or six times before moving round to the other side of the body.

FRONT OF LEGS

EFFLEURAGE

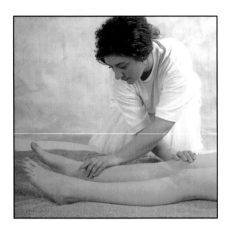

Apply oil to both legs using an effleurage movement working up from the ankles, as used on the back of the legs.

Repeat the effleurage strokes sequence several times to ensure an even distribution of oil.

LEG STRETCH

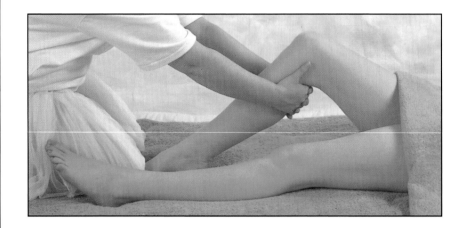

Supporting the leg at the ankle and behind the knee, bend the leg up and place it in line with the shoulder.

Clasp the hands around the back of the knee. Ask your partner to inhale deeply, then pull the calf muscle toward you.

Hold for a slow count of three. As your partner breathes out, release the pull on the calf.

Repeat the whole movement three times, then gently lay the leg down and repeat the stretch on the other leg.

ARMS AND HANDS

EFFLEURAGE

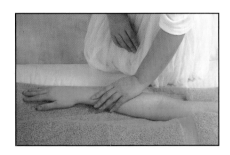

1 *Seated to the side of your partner, move the arm slightly away from the body. Apply the oil by sweeping from just above the wrist, up to the shoulder and round.*

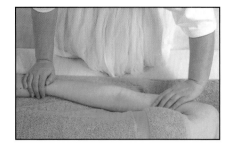

2 *As the first hand comes off the arm, the other hand starts at the wrist and sweeps upward to the gland sited in the elbow joint.*

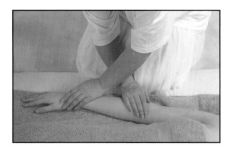

3 *The first arm crosses the second as it reaches the elbow and again sweeps from wrist to shoulder.*

Repeat six or seven times.

You can follow the effleurage *with flushing to the inside*
of the arm, using the same movements performed on the leg, working
from the wrist to the elbow.
Before going on to the second arm, massage the hand of the first arm.

HAND MASSAGE

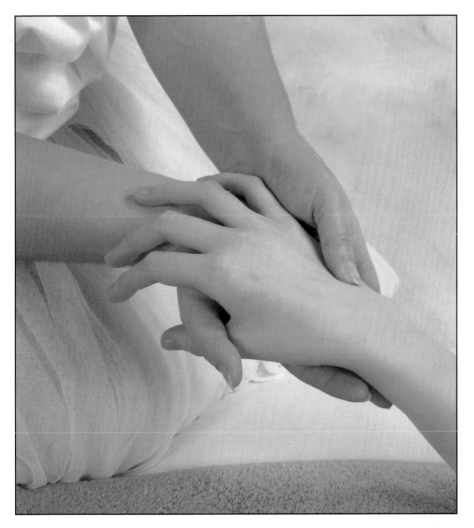

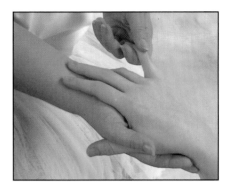

2 *Pull back to the fingers, gently*
massaging the joints between
your thumb and forefinger as you
draw towards the tips. Finish with
a slight pull to the finger to stretch
it out.

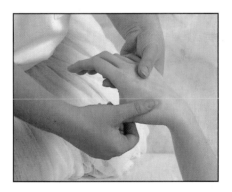

1 *Resting your partner's hand*
palm down over your own
palm, use small brushing

movements with your thumbs to
work upward between the joints of
the fingers toward the wrist.

3 *Repeat with each finger,*
finishing with the thumb.

Now repeat the movements on the other arm and hand.

To finish the massage, cover your partner to the neck, check he or she
is warm and comfortable, and leave to rest for a minimum of five minutes (up to
15 minutes is preferable). Upon returning, help your partner to sit up
carefully and offer a glass of water.

PREGNANCY TREATMENTS

Pregnancy can be one of the most exciting and fulfilling times of a woman's life. The joy of bringing another human being into the world creates a tremendous feeling of contentment and anticipation, but it is also a time of great physical and emotional upheaval. Together with the ever-important trio of exercise, good diet and rest, essential oils can play an important role in helping a woman cope with the stresses of nine months of pregnancy, the pain of labour and post-natal recovery.

COMMON AILMENTS

Surging hormone levels and changes in your swelling body can bring a host of discomforts, many of which can be alleviated by aromatherapy treatments and other simple steps.

Backache
The lower back region takes a lot of strain during pregnancy, and will benefit from a firm massage with four drops each of lavender and sandalwood in two tablespoons of base oil. Six drops of lavender in the bath will help to soothe away the aches.

Morning Sickness
Eat little and often during the day, avoiding junk food and heavy meals late at night. Choose fresh foods which are free from preservatives or chemicals. Try herbal tea infusions such as chamomile, peppermint or orange blossom, which are good for the digestion.

Heartburn
Avoid heavy meals and particularly rich, spicy foods. Peppermint tea infusions help, and you can rub the solar plexus with a blend of two drops each of lemon and peppermint essential oils in one tablespoon of base oil.

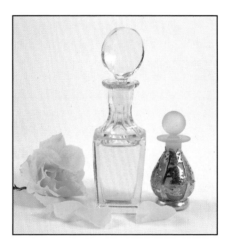

Spoil yourself with the luxurious and relaxing scent of rose for body and facial oils, to keep your spirits up during pregnancy.

Sore Breasts
These need extra care and attention during pregnancy as they expand. Use a gentle massage oil with rose and orange, three drops of each in one tablespoon of sweet almond oil; or if breasts are swollen, make a cool compress using rosewater and place over the breasts while having an afternoon rest. Sweet almond oil on its own is excellent for sore, cracked nipples during breast-feeding. Never use pure essential oils on the breasts during this period as they can easily be transferred to the baby while feeding.

Constipation
Make sure your diet contains plenty of fresh and high fibre foods and drink plenty of still water. Tension can also be a contributory factor, so try a relaxing bath with three drops of lavender and four drops of rose. Massage your abdomen and the small of the back with a blend of four drops of chamomile or orange in one tablespoon of base oil.

Sleep Problems
In the last few months of pregnancy, with the baby kicking and other discomforts, it is often difficult to get a good night's sleep. A relaxing bath with neroli and rose is soothing, and you can add ylang-ylang for its calming, sedative effect – a maximum of eight drops in total. Two drops of rose or lavender on the edge of the pillowcase will help induce sleep.

Stretch Marks
When the stretched skin returns to the body's normal shape it can leave tiny jagged scars. A daily massage around the hips and expanding tummy, using five drops of lavender in one tablespoon of jojoba, wheatgerm or evening primrose oil, will help keep skin smooth and supple. Start around the fifth month of

pregnancy and continue after the birth until you return to your normal weight.

Swollen Ankles
These can be reduced with a cool to warm footbath of benzoin, rose and orange. Add two drops of each directly to the bowl or mix with one tablespoon of base carrier oil such as sesame seed. Rest with feet raised on cushions or pillows.

Varicose Veins
During pregnancy the blood flow to the legs is often slowed down, causing the veins to dilate. Two drops each of cypress, lemongrass and lavender, mixed with two tablespoons of apricot kernel base oil, can be smoothed gently over the legs for relief. If veins are prominent then one of the best oils for the circulation is geranium, though this should always be very dilute for use in pregnancy. Add four drops to the bath or to one tablespoon of carrier oil to massage the leg with upward movements. Do not work directly on the veins or apply too much pressure to the leg.

LABOUR

To create a relaxing atmosphere in the labour room, use a few drops of lavender in a fragrancer, or try rose, neroli or ylang-ylang to fortify you as the labour progresses. Any of these oils can be used in a massage blend for the lower back to help with contractions. If labour is progressing slowly, try marjoram as a massage oil or compress across the abdomen to stimulate contractions.

AFTER THE BIRTH

The "baby blues" often occur around the third or fourth day after childbirth, though some

CAUTIONS

The following oils should be avoided during pregnancy (particularly the first five months) because of their strong diuretic properties or tendency to induce menstruation:

Bay · Basil · Clary Sage · Comfrey Fennel · Hyssop · Juniper Marjoram · Melissa · Myrrh Rosemary · Thyme · Sage

Use all essential oils in half the usual quantity during pregnancy and take extra care in handling them. Ensure that the oils you are using are pure essential oils, as adulterated blends or synthetic oils can sometimes have less predictable effects.

If you have a history of miscarriage you could also avoid chamomile and lavender for the first few months, although in general these are excellent oils for pregnancy.

Because of their potentially toxic nature and strong abortive qualities the following oils should *never* be used except by a qualified aromatherapist, and must be avoided during pregnancy:

Oreganum · Pennyroyal · St John's Wort · Tansy · Wormwood

women can suffer a more severe form of post-natal depression for up to a year. A bath of jasmine and ylang-ylang will help you feel better, or use a body oil of chamomile, geranium and orange (5 drops to two tablespoons of sweet almond oil), which is a good mix for hormonal imbalance.

To ease any perineal pains, a bath with lavender is soothing. Tea tree can also be added, since this is a powerful antiseptic and helps heal internal wounds and stitches.

Recommended Oils for Pregnancy
Chamomile · Geranium (in low doses) *· Lavender · Lemon · Neroli Orange · Rose · Sandalwood*

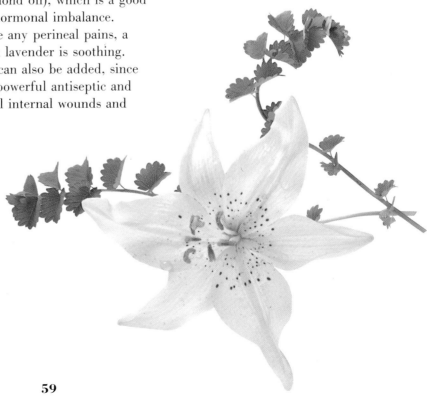

PREGNANCY MASSAGE

These simple touch massage movements can help to relieve many of the stresses and discomforts of pregnancy, and the back massage is particularly welcome during labour. The basic essential oil massage is modified in various ways to take account of the pregnant condition.

- Check the box on the previous page to find which oils are suitable and which are to be avoided.
- Use a lower concentration of essential oil to base oil; $^{1}/_{2}$–1 per cent is ideal.
- Keep strokes lighter than usual.
- In addition to the steps suggested, you can incorporate a facial and gentle breast massage.
- It is particularly important to observe the rest period after the massage and to help your partner get up gently.
- The positions you work in need to be adapted for a pregnant woman, as she cannot lie out straight on her front or back and needs to be well supported.

THE BACK

After about the fourth month of pregnancy it becomes uncomfortable to lie on the stomach, so work with your partner sitting up with a towel-wrapped pillow or back of a chair to lean over for support.

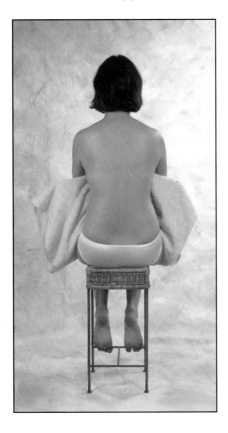

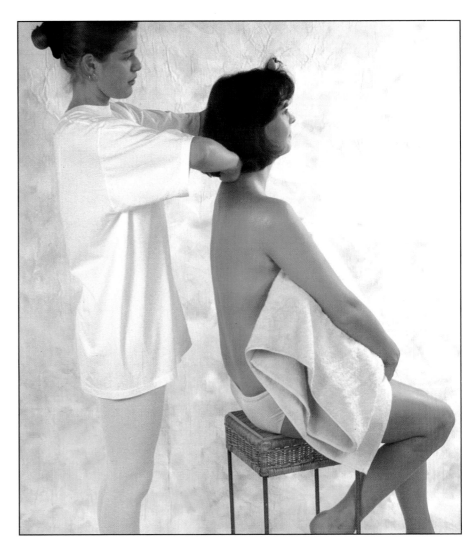

1 *Make sure your partner is comfortable and place your left hand over the forehead and the palm of your right hand across the back of the neck. Hold for a few moments and then release.*

60

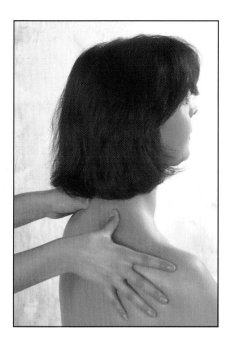

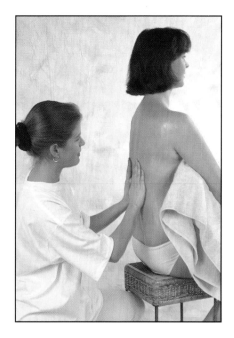

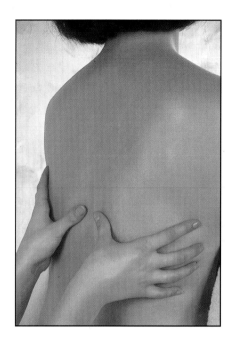

2 *Apply a little oil to your fingers and using a slight but gentle pressure, softly massage each side of your partner's neck and shoulders, kneading mainly with the thumbs. This will help to relieve the tension often caused by the weight of enlarged breasts.*

3 *Stroke the oil evenly over the back and begin an effleurage movement (a soothing, stroking motion with two hands, moving up the sides of the spine and out over the shoulders). Repeat several times to establish a rhythm and relax your partner.*

4 *Using the thumbs, work upward on each side of the spinal column from the lower back to the neck to help release congestion along the spinal nerves. Repeat four times. Clear the movement by sweeping up the back using the calming effleurage stroke.*

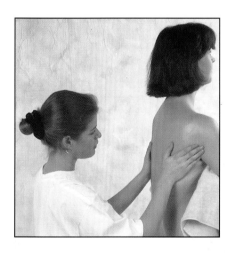

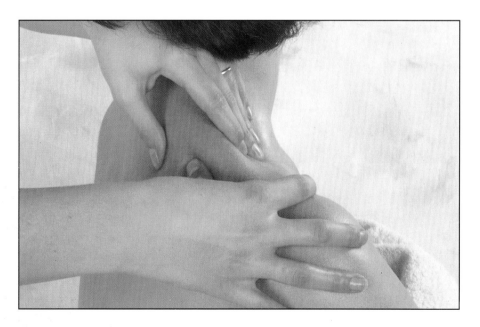

5 *Starting from the centre of the back, begin working up and outward across the width of the back with superficial effleurage movements. Repeat the movements several times until your partner is relaxed. This will help to stimulate the circulation and has a soothing effect on the nerve endings.*

6 *Using a double-handed movement, press down and then gently lift the muscles to the side of the neck, rolling with the thumb, and then release. Work out* *from the neck across the shoulder, and then repeat across the other shoulder. Performed slowly with rhythmic movements this is very relaxing and will alleviate stiffness.*

THE ABDOMEN

For a pregnant woman, the weight of the uterus can constrict important blood vessels if she lies down flat on her back, so provide plenty of pillows, cushions, bolsters or rolled towels to support your partner behind the back, under the neck and knees and anywhere else she needs to feel comfortable.

1 *Below: It may seem alarming to massage the abdomen during pregnancy but, providing the strokes are light and careful, it is safe and relaxing for mother and baby. Gentle massage all over the abdominal area can be very soothing and is beneficial for relieving the stretched feeling often experienced during pregnancy. Apply oil evenly over the area to help feed the tissues and lessen the possibility of stretch marks.*

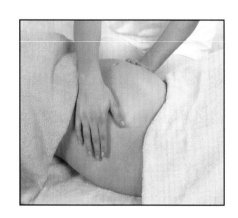

2 *Using the flat of your hands, carefully glide them up from either side of the waist, lifting your hands off as they reach the navel, and then start again. Continue to stroke the area with a light, soft touch, working over the whole of the abdomen to soothe and calm.*

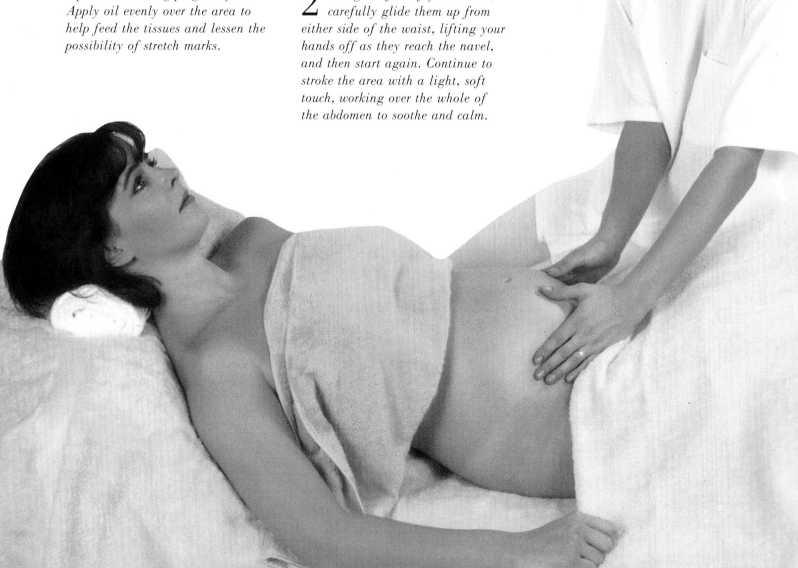

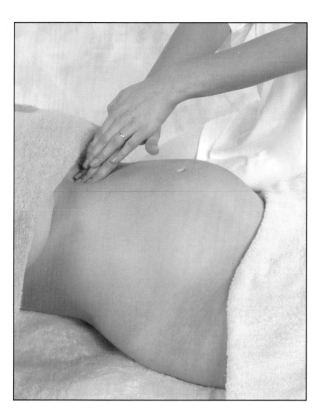

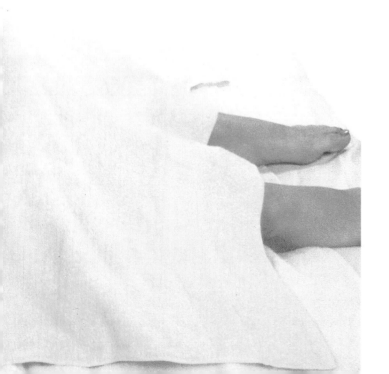

3 *After a minute of gentle circular movements, place the fingertips of your left hand on the higher section of the solar plexus region and cover with your right hand. Rest both hands for a moment and then release to help alleviate stress.*

LEGS

Make sure your partner is comfortable, with the knees supported by cushions.

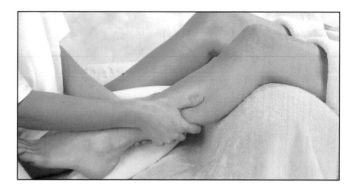

Begin gently stroking the leg with an effleurage *from the ankle to the knee, smoothing up the shin and then glide around the calf.*
It can help to relieve the swelling, varicose veins or cramp which afflict many pregnant women. Do not use any heavy movements to the legs and avoid any reflexology movements to the feet, though gentle stroking around the ankles may well be appreciated.

TO FINISH

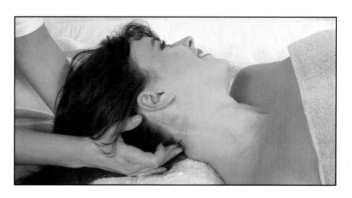

With both hands positioned at the back of the neck, apply light circular pressures to the cranium (skull) with your fingertips working in an upward direction to help release tension.

End the massage by smoothing the hair away from the neck and forehead, releasing all the negative energy. Allow your partner to rest for 15 minutes and then help her to get up very gently.

BEAUTY BASICS

Looking good starts with great skin, and aromatherapy can help you achieve this in various ways: the remarkable penetrative properties of essential oils make them excellent moisturizers, and the wide range of their properties means there is always the right oil for the right condition. For instance, rosemary stimulates the circulation and thyme help the cells to regenerate. As well as being stimulating to the lymphatic system, which helps cleanse the tissue that causes sluggish skin, essential oils can be used as part of your daily skin-care routine and to treat specific problems such as acne.

FEED YOUR SKIN

Skin needs to be fed and nourished – inside and out. Healthy diets can keep the body in shape but to keep skin in peak condition it needs to have a ready supply of valuable vitamins and minerals. Many factors can drain the body of this valuable resource – canned and over-processed foods, caffeine, alcohol, nicotine, sunlight, central heating, carbon monoxide and habitual drug taking. The effects of these can build up and attack the skin so from time to time you need to give it a break.

A one-day fruit and vegetable diet is an excellent regime to adopt once a month to cleanse your body and give a boost to your system.

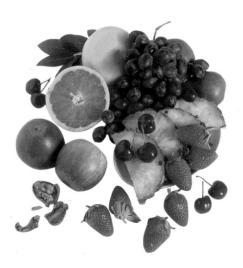

SKIN TYPES

Choose the right oils for your skin type and use them to blend your own cleansers, toners, masks and moisturizing facial oils. Remember that skin types can vary: skin may be drier in winter or summer or more prone to oiliness around the time of your period, and it can change several times between puberty and menopause. So review the oils you use to suit your skin now and vary them to meet the changing needs of your complexion.

Few people are blessed with normal skin and even those who are may tend towards dryness or oiliness at times. Letters in parentheses indicate what other skin types an oil is suitable for. D = dry, S = sensitive, O = oily, A = all skin types.

Oils for Normal Skin
Chamomile (D, S) · Fennel (O) Geranium (A) · Lavender (A) Lemon (O) · Patchouli (D) Rose (D, S) · Sandalwood (D, S)

Oils for Dry Skin
Chamomile · Geranium · Lavender Hyssop · Rose · Patchouli Sandalwood · Ylang-Ylang

Oils for Sensitive Skin
Chamomile · Lavender · Neroli Rose · Sandalwood

Oils for Oily Skin
Bergamot · Cedarwood · Cypress Lavender · Lemon · Geranium Juniper · Frankincense · Sage

Combination skin has an oily T-zone panel from the forehead down to the nose and chin area, and may be normal or dry elsewhere. Double up on the treatments, using oils for oily skin on the greasy patches and oils for normal skin on the rest of the face area.

CLEANSERS

Choose the correct essential oils for your skin type and blend them in with an ordinary unperfumed brand of cleanser, liquid soap, or tissue-off lotion/cream, and they will do nature's work of rebalancing the skin.

FACIAL STEAM

Add five drops of chamomile for a soothing steam or try lavender, peppermint, thyme or rosemary to stimulate; comfrey or fennel for their healing properties.

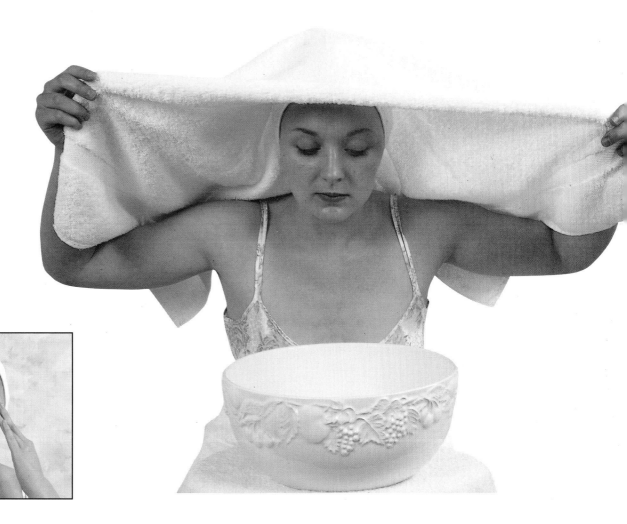

Above: Cleanse the face, paying particular attention to the oilier areas.

Above right: For a facial steam, boil the water, cool slightly and add the oils. Steam for five minutes.

TONERS

Essential oils are the gentlest way of toning up. Rose water for normal or dry/sensitive skin or witchhazel for oilier skins are ideal bases for fresheners. These can be applied with cotton wool or for a more refreshing tone, sprayed on to the face.

Herbal tea infusions are also ideal toners. Boil a cup of water and infuse chamomile, marigold, rosehip or nettle teas (you can use herbal tea bags if you can't get hold of the herbs), add two drops of orange or lavender oil and leave to cool. Oily skin benefits from juniper or lemongrass whereas drier skins would appreciate rose or sandalwood.

FACIAL OILS

Well-moisturized skin is soft and supple, reflects a healthy glow and ages less quickly. Younger skin only needs light conditioning whereas older skin needs specific nourishing treatments. Most moisturizers soothe and sit on the surface of the skin, but essential oils, with their fine molecular structure, work their way through from the surface to the inner dermis (the skin's deeper regenerating layer). Mixed with the correct amount of base oil, these pure essentials do not clog up pores on lubrication: they are light enough to be absorbed spontaneously by skin.

Use two tablespoons of base oil and add six drops of essential oil (maximum of three different oils) to suit individual needs.

MASKS

Both clay and oatmeal are ideal ingredients for any face mask. A natural powdered clay is fuller's earth, which can be mixed into a paste with hot water. Cool and then add yogurt for a smoother consistency. Similarly, finely ground oatmeal can be mixed into a paste and left to cool. Add 15 drops of essential oils to suit your skin type per cupful of paste. Smooth on to your face, leave to dry slightly and then sponge off. For particularly dry/sensitive skins add one tablespoon evening primrose base oil to give a more moisturizing mask. When applying, avoid the eye area.

EYE TREATS

While relaxing with a face mask on, close the eyes and cover with cotton pads soaked in rose water, or soothe with two slices of fresh cucumber.

ACNE

Because of their anti-bacterial, anti-inflammatory and rebalancing properties, essential oils are ideal skin treatments for acne sufferers.

It is often a mistake to scrub oily skin over-zealously: this only activates the sebaceous glands which in turn produce more sebum. If you suffer from pustular acne then avoid excessive facial steams which may spread the condition: use a mask instead. Often it is better to opt for a daily sensitive-skin type cleanser and moisturizer, adding two drops of juniper, which is stimulating and antiseptic. Opt for a deeper clay-type mask treatment once a week, adding a couple of drops of juniper, which is healing, soothing and tightening, or eucalyptus which is anti-inflammatory, antiseptic and antibiotic. Increase your intake of vitamin E, which is a great skin healer.

BROKEN VEINS

These small, red, spider-like thread veins often appear on the surface of skin around the cheek area. They are broken capillaries and seem to affect those with a delicate or fragile skin type. Hot and cold elements, along with stimulants such as alcohol and caffeine, can often trigger this condition. To treat it at home the secret is to protect the skin from losing excess moisture and to give it extra essential oil treatments using parsley, geranium, chamomile, rosemary or cypress in a heavy base oil.

COLD SORES

Cold sores are small blisters on the lips or surrounding area which are caused by the virus herpes simplex. It normally lies dormant in nerve cells but can surface following a simple cold or flu. Any lip sore that persists should be treated medically but for the common cold sore a dab of undiluted tea tree oil will help.

ODD SPOTS

If prone to occasional spots then mix one drop each of neroli, lemon and lavender in one teaspoon (5 ml) of base oil and treat just the affected area. For a single spot use a cotton bud and dab on one drop of undiluted sandalwood.

FACIAL MASSAGE

Massage helps the skin to absorb oils and creams easily.
Give skin a clear start with our step-by-step facial.

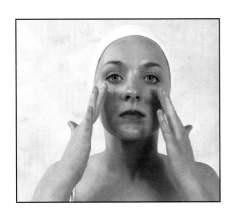

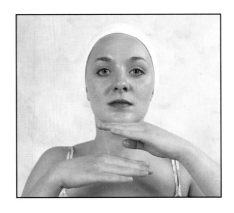

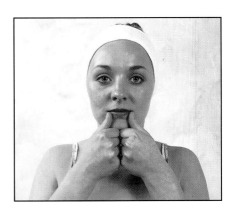

1 *Pour a small amount of blended oil into the palm of your hand and gently apply all over the face, avoiding the eyes.*

2 *With the back of your hands, gently tap the skin around the jaw-line and underneath the chin to stimulate the skin cells.*

3 *Apply small circular movements to the chin area, using your thumbs, to tone, help circulation and eliminate toxins.*

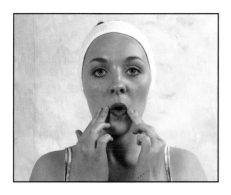

4 *Make an "oooh"-shaped mouth. Massage either side easing out fine lines.*

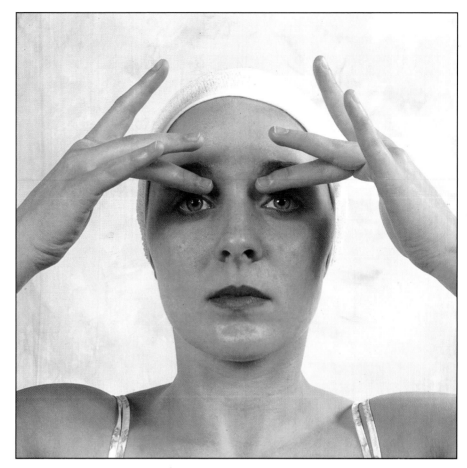

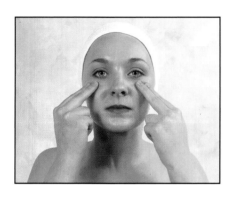

5 *With your fingertips, press along the top of the cheekbones and massage outward up to the temples to release toxins.*

6 *With the middle fingers, apply pressure to points above the bridge of the nose and underneath the eyebrows. Hold for five seconds* and smooth across from the inner to the outer corners of the eyebrows and continue up to the temples.

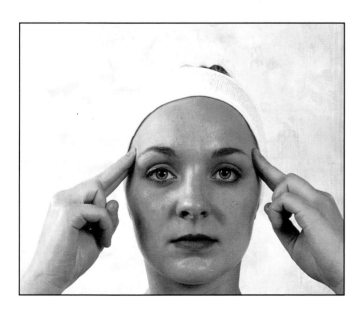

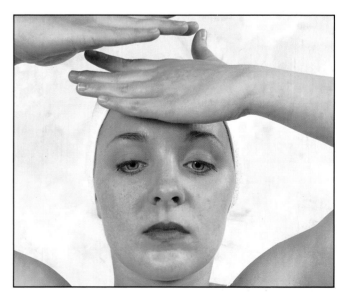

7 *To relieve tension, apply firm pressure at either side of the temples, and rotate backward.*

8 *Stroke up the forehead to the hairline with the palms of the hands, smoothing out fine lines.*

HEALTHY HAIR

Hair can define your image and style but it is also a mirror of your health. Emotional or physical problems can soon result in a lack of bounce or shine.

Keeping hair in peak condition is a combination of caring for it on the surface and nurturing it from inside with a well-balanced diet.

SCALP MASSAGE OILS

Dry hair is rough to touch, thick in texture and dries out at the first sign of heated rollers or tongs. Avoid chemical colourants and perms and opt for shampoos and conditioners with jojoba and almond oils. Hot oil treatments allow essential oils to soak in easily and condition the hair. After massaging warm oil into the scalp, wrap the head in a warm towel and leave on for half an hour.

Oils for Dry Hair
Rose · Sandalwood · Ylang-ylang Lavender · Geranium

Greasy hair tends to look dull, lank, lacks body and won't hold a style. Central heating and environmental elements aggravate the condition but it can stem from a hormonal imbalance. Check your diet and avoid harsh degreasing shampoos. Clean brushes and combs weekly. Plastic brushes are better for brushing through as bristle continually stimulates the scalp. Choose light conditioning rinses to detangle but try a scalp massage to regulate the oil-producing sebaceous glands.

Oils for Greasy Hair
Basil · Eucalyptus · Cedarwood Chamomile · Lemongrass Cypress · Sage · Rosemary

Normal hair is glossy with plenty of natural body and bounce. An occasional hot-oil scalp treatment

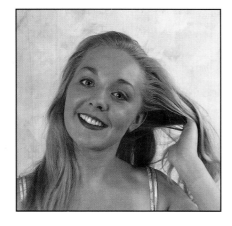

will keep it looking good and growing healthily.

Oils for Normal Hair
Geranium · Lavender Lemongrass · Rosemary

Combination hair has ends that are dry or normal and the roots are greasy. Avoid using hot appliances near the scalp and keep the ends regularly trimmed and conditioned. Use a scalp treatment with oils for greasy hair but don't comb through to the ends.

How to Mix
Base oils Choose from sweet almond, apricot kernal, avocado, jojoba, evening primrose or sunflower.

Essential oils For one scalp treatment, choose up to three oils and use five drops of each for two tablespoons of base oil (for very long hair you may need more oil). Warm the blended oils by placing the container in a bowl of boiling water, and then massage into the scalp. Wrap with a hot towel, leave for 15 minutes and then shampoo.

HAIR PROBLEMS

Dandruff
There are two types: dry and the more common oily. It's not catching! It can be caused by factors such as chemical body changes, stress, poor eating habits or wrong application of hair products. Both flakey and dry scalps can be treated with essential oils. Use special dandruff shampoos and conditioning rinses and treat the scalp by gently massaging with oils to suit. Use a base oil formula with patchouli and tea tree. For a dry, itchy scalp try cedarwood and lavender.

Grey Hair
Grey hair is more porous and needs extra conditioning, particularly if it is chemically treated or coloured. Use a scalp formula for dry hair adding essential oil enhancers like chamomile to lighten or sage to darken any discolouration.

Hair Loss
Hair coming out in handfuls is often due to a hormonal imbalance, stress or anxiety, so the first step is to learn to relax. Any unusual thinning patch should be looked at by a trichologist but, as a general remedy, use a scalp massage with lavender and rosemary oils.

SCALP MASSAGE

This is a wonderful way to condition hair, stimulate the scalp and relieve tension. You can use these steps to treat your own hair but it's even more relaxing if you can persuade a friend to help, especially if you've got long hair.

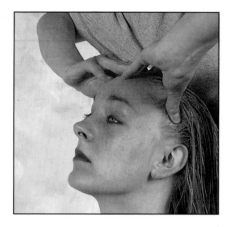

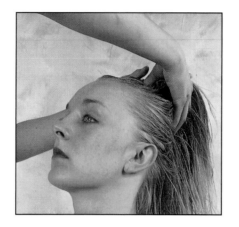

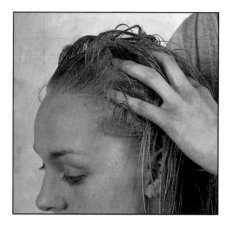

1 *Shampoo the hair and towel dry to absorb excess water. Comb through with a wide-tooth comb. Tilt your head back and pour some oil on to the hairline, massaging in with thumbs on the temple and fingers spread apart over the centre of the head.*

2 *Loosely run fingers and oil over the top of the scalp from front to back, lifting hair at the crown. Keep dipping your fingertips in the treatment oil to spread through the hair while massaging.*

3 *Massage the head with kneading movements. Grip and push (with fingerpads, rather than fingernails) against the scalp. The scalp should gently rotate against the skull. Concentrate on one area at a time, with the hands positioned on either side of the scalp.*

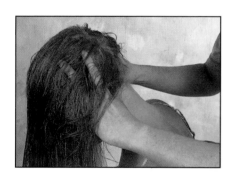

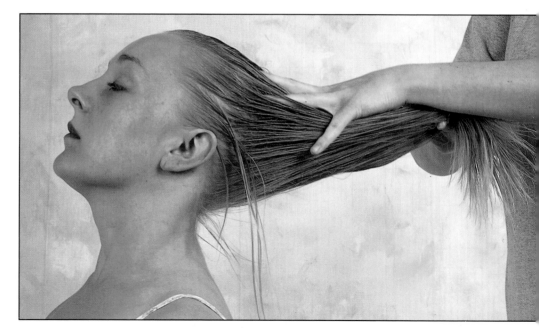

4 *Scalp massage works from front to back, from the forehead, frontal hairline, temples and sides, over the crown of the head to the base of the neck, following the natural flow of blood. If the scalp feels particularly tight then concentrate on areas where the scalp doesn't want to move. At the base of the skull, press firmly and push the whole scalp up toward the crown to release tension.*

5 *Pull any extra oil through the hair, working out from the roots to the tips. Make sure all the hair is well oiled, and then leave towel-wrapped for at least 15 minutes before shampooing.*

THE AROMATIC BATH

The relaxing and remedial properties of water and of massaging oils into the body were recognized in ancient Greek and Roman cultures, when bathing first became a daily ritual.

A bath with essential oils is one of the simplest and most effective aromatherapy treatments. It can be stimulating or relaxing, depending on the temperature of the water and whether you choose oils with uplifting or calming properties. In the bath, the therapeutic action of the oils is two-fold: they are absorbed through the skin, moisturizing the dermis and entering the circulatory system, and at the same time their aromas are inhaled, stimulating the brain and increasing your sense of well-being. An aromatic bath can detoxify the body, help problems like cellulite, joint stiffness, general aches and pains, colds and headaches, tone and condition skin, and relieve anxiety and tension.

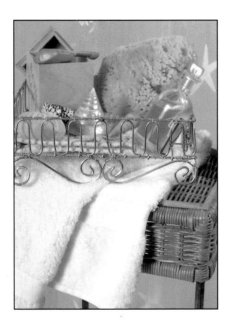

RUNNING THE BATH

Bath temperature and the time spent in the tub are important. A cooler bath is more stimulating and warmer water relaxes. Very hot water is damaging, however: it causes blood vessels and capillaries to expand and increases the heart beat. You should particularly avoid hot water if you have varicose veins, haemorrhoids, high blood pressure or are pregnant. A 15–20 minute soak is long enough before skin cells over-hydrate and swell with water. Wait until the bath is almost full before adding the oils, as they evaporate so quickly.

OILS FOR THE BATH

Essential oils are the best way of making a bath both aromatic and therapeutic. They sink into the skin easily and at the same time impart their lovely herbal or floral fragrances. You can add drops of oil directly to the bath and they will float on the surface in a fine film and evaporate, giving you the full benefit of their aromas. Or if you want to absorb them more you can disperse them through the water by mixing with a base carrier oil such as sweet almond, apricot kernel, jojoba or evening primrose (these rich base oils all nourish and rejuvenate the skin in their own right).

Mix a bath oil with a combination of up to three essential oils, five drops from each, in one tablespoon of skin-softening base oil. Choose oils with similar or complementary effects so they do not counter-balance one another.

THE RELAXING BATH

To calm yourself after a fraught day or to prepare yourself for a peaceful night's sleep, turn your bathroom into a private sanctuary. Keep the light soft if possible, or use an eye mask or burn aromatic candles. Plants create an oxygenated atmosphere. Support your head with a bath pillow, close your eyes and inhale deeply. Concentrate on your breathing, empty your mind and let the oils soothe away the stresses and strains. After a 15–20 minute soak, get out slowly and wrap yourself in a large, warm towel.

Oils for Relaxation
Basil · Bergamot · Cedarwood Chamomile · Frankincense Hyssop · Juniper · Lavender Marjoram · Melissa · Neroli Patchouli · Rose · Sage Sandalwood · Ylang-Ylang

Although these oils have a predominantly calming effect some can also be used to stimulate the circulation and lymphatic system, in particular lavender oil and also bergamot.

THE STIMULATING BATH

Best for the morning to get you started or to revive you before an evening out. Keep the water fairly cool and use an invigorating bath mitt to rub down and stimulate the circulation. When you've soaked, rinse yourself with water as cold as you can bear, either by splashing directly from the tap (faucet) or shower, or by adding more cold water to cool down your bath.

As you get out, either slap yourself dry to make the skin tingle or rub yourself vigorously with a towel.

Oils for Stimulation
Cypress · Eucalyptus · Fennel Geranium · Juniper · Lavender Lemon · Lemongrass · Peppermint Pine · Rosemary · Thyme

THERAPEUTIC BATHS

Oils for Dermatitis
Chamomile · Hyssop · Lavender
Oils for Eczema
Chamomile · Geranium · Hyssop Juniper · Rosemary · Myrrh
Oils for Psoriasis
Bergamot · Chamomile · Lavender
Oils for Arthritis/Rheumatism
Chamomile · Eucalyptus · Juniper Lavender · Rosemary · Thyme

SHOWERS AND COLD RINSES

nvigorating jets of water are ideal for getting the blood pumping and there's no need to forego the benefits of aromatic oils. Skin tends to be sluggish in the cold winter months but sloughing off dead top layers can help regenerate cells and allow moisturizers to be absorbed more easily. Showers are ideal for smoothing skin with exfoliating rubs using wet salt, a loofah or a mitt to slough off the top surface of dead skin cells. A dry friction glove or loofah is too harsh for most skins so soften first in warm water. Soft bristle brushes can also help to get the circulation going with gentle massage on problem areas like hips and thighs. To keep friction brushes and mitts fresh always rinse and hang up to dry.

Essential oils can be used under the shower: try a base oil mixed with invigorating essences and with a clean face-cloth or sponge, pour on the oils and rub all over the body in circular motions whilst showering. To clear the sinuses and help coughs and colds, sponge the chest with a mix of eucalyptus and peppermint oils. A cold-water shower after cleansing improves the circulation and tightens skin pores.

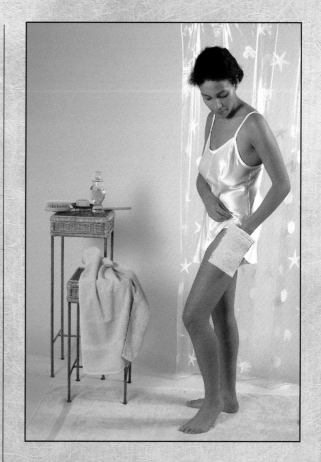

Start off your shower or bath routine by whisking off dead skin cells with a friction mitt. Moisten the palm of the mitt with warm water or softening oils such as sweet almond or evening primrose. Concentrate on outer thighs, working from the knee in upward circular movements across the buttocks.

AFTER-BATH BODY TREATMENTS

Moisturizing oils and lotions applied after the bath or shower help to nourish the skin, keeping it soft and supple. As we get older our skin dehydrates since the oil glands do not produce as much oil as in youth.

Apply a body oil all over the body, starting from the feet and working right up to the neck and tips of the ears. Avoid talcum powders which clog the pores and tend to have a drying effect.

BODY-OIL FORMULA

Essential oils sink beautifully into warm damp skin. For a lasting effect, mix the three chosen bath essential oils, five drops of each, in two tablespoons of base oil. If you want to make up a larger quantity of body oil, use a concentration of three per cent essential oil in base oil.

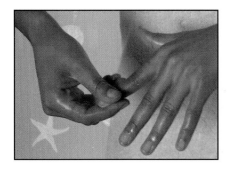

Above: Condition hands and nails with a simple finger-pulling exercise. Spread and stretch the fingers straight out; massage each finger with oils, working from the tip of the nails to the cuticles and up to each finger knuckle.

Right: Soften the feet after a bath by massaging between the toes and then working around the tougher skin and heel areas. Finish with sweeping movements all over to stimulate the circulation.

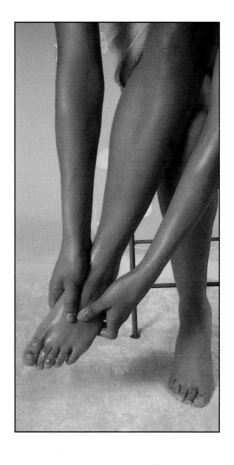

PROBLEM ZONES

Hands and nails take some rough treatment with everyday chores. The ideal time for a manicure or pedicure is after soaking in a bath when nails and skin are softened, making it easy to clean around the nail bed and to clip uneven nails without snagging.

Fragile or flakey nails benefit from a rich, nourishing treatment: rub them with apricot kernel, wheatgerm or jojoba oil. Restore hands with a soothing, moisturizing mix of one tablespoon of sweet almond oil and five drops each of patchouli, lavender and lemon.

Feet are often neglected until they hurt. Polish hard skin around heels and soles with a handful of damp salt or use a pumice stone. While in the bath, bend one knee, grip the toes and then work with the fingers massaging in an upward direction, from the toes to the heels and up the calves in order to stimulate blood flow and relax tired feet. Massage a body oil into the feet after a bath, shower or pedicure.

For a deodorizing and soothing footbath add three drops each of cypress and lavender to a basin full of water. Chilblains can be treated with a massage blend of three drops of geranium and a drop each of lavender and rosemary in one tablespoon of sweet almond base oil.

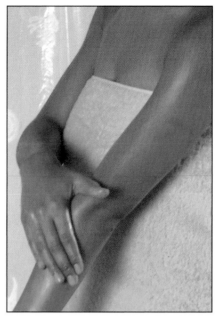

Above: Apply body oil to the arms with smooth upward strokes, concentrating on the elbows and upper arms where the skin is often rougher and drier.

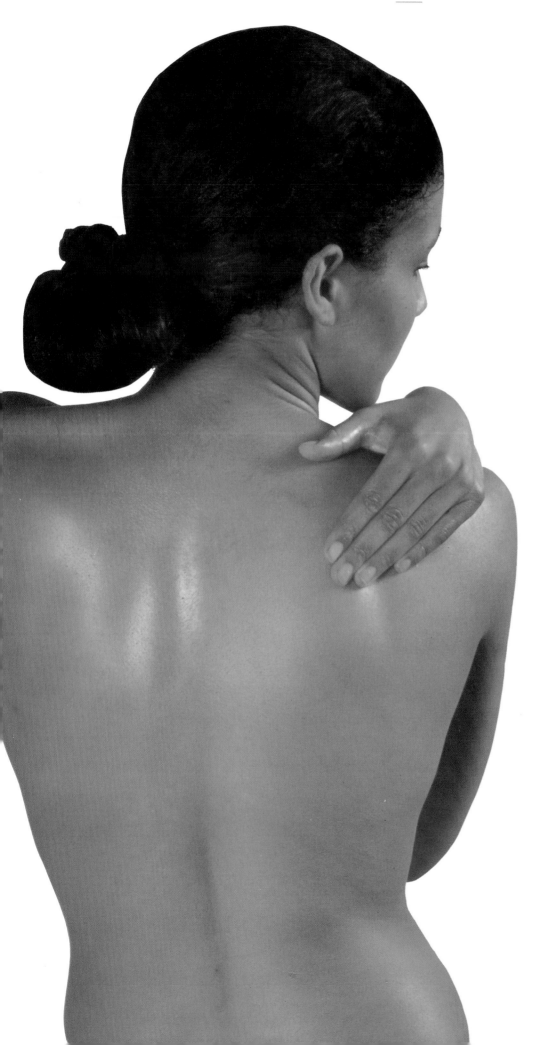

Elbows can soon build up hard protective layers of grey, unsightly skin. A good softener for tough elbows is a sweet almond oil and oatmeal scrub. Mix three tablespoons of sweet almond oil with three tablespoons of fine oatmeal and mix to a paste with fresh milk or yoghurt. Smooth and rub over the elbows and any grey, goosey areas of skin around upper arms. Add six drops of fennel if arms are flabby. Another great elbow booster is the traditional recipe of cutting a lemon in half, squeezing out the juice and rubbing the elbows in the hollow of the lemon.

Left: When it comes to applying body oil, the back, neck and shoulders are often neglected because they are difficult to reach, but these are key areas for releasing tension and the skin needs to be nourished, so smooth as far as possible, or enlist the help of a friend.

IN THE REALM OF THE SENSES

The power of perfume to inspire romance has been known since the Babylonians, and perfume and flowers are still today the favourite gifts for lovers. Cleopatra's seduction of Mark Antony was carefully staged with a carpet of rose petals and rare and exotic scents in every conceivable form – even the sails of her barge were drenched in perfume to catch the breeze and announce her arrival.

The sense of smell is fundamental to our sensuality. Pheromones, chemicals secreted in human sweat, act as the most basic trigger to sexual attraction. The smells of flowers and plants are the plant equivalent of pheromones, irresistible to birds and bees and just as attractive to humans. We can use natural aromatic plant oils to relax, heighten our awareness, excite the senses and create a mood for love.

SETTING THE SCENE

Create a calming and sensual atmosphere with scented candles or a few drops of essential oil evaporated in a fragrancer or light-bulb ring. Dim the lights and turn up the heat.

Scent your lingerie or bedlinen by adding three drops of your favourite oil to the final rinse, or store them in drawers with aromatic bags or scented balls. Sprinkle drops of rose or jasmine on the pillows.

PREPARING YOUR BODY

Luxuriate in an aromatic bath or hot tub, or, better still, share it with your partner. After soaking, perfume your whole body with a rich body oil or use a strong concentration to dab pulse points such as wrists, temples and behind the ears and knees, and wait for your partner to discover these secret scented areas.

PARTNER MASSAGE

We are all sensual beings and yet at times we may need help to switch off from everyday concerns and tune in to our senses. The loving touch of partner massage is always enjoyable; it is relaxing and yet sensually stimulating – a total physical experience.

You can adapt the basic essential massage, using plenty of *effleurage* all over, deeper kneading for tense areas and light feather strokes with the fingertips to excite the surface of the skin. Avoid the lymph drainage movements as these are distinctly unerotic! Discover your partner's erogenous zones – explore the ears and feet and the inside of the forearms and thighs. Find some more. Be tender and loving, playful and creative – let your imagination guide you.

OILS FOR SEDUCTION

Most of the aphrodisiac oils combine well with each other, but be careful not to use too many together or they may clash and work against each other. Subtlety is the key to the art of seduction.

- *Clary sage* – sweet, sensuous and slightly intoxicating, but be careful as in high doses its sedative effect will inhibit sex drive.
- *Geranium* – a strong floral that both relaxes and uplifts.
- *Jasmine* – the heady floral fragrance boosts confidence and creates a luxurious atmosphere.
- *Neroli* – fresh and sweet, its fortifying effect helps overcome shyness and inhibitions.
- *Patchouli* – heavy and exotic, it is stimulating in small doses and heightens the senses.
- *Rose* – the quintessential oil for lovers. Rare and powerful.
- *Sandalwood* – woody, sweet and exotic with spicy undertones.
- *Ylang-Ylang* – the long-lasting floral scent gives a feeling of relaxed well-being, helpful for impotence or frigidity.

You can also try the warm, spicy exotics such as black pepper, ginger, cardamon, cinnamon or cedarwood, but be sparing with these as they can easily overpower.

Layer the scents by choosing just three or four and using them in different strengths and combinations for the room fragrance, bath, body oil or massage blend.

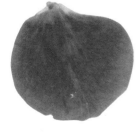

With a massage oil blended from floral and spicy aphrodisiac essences you can arouse the intimate senses of touch and smell simultaneously as you explore the skin and curves of your partner's body with strong smoothing strokes. Let the heady scents work their spell on the senses and emotions.

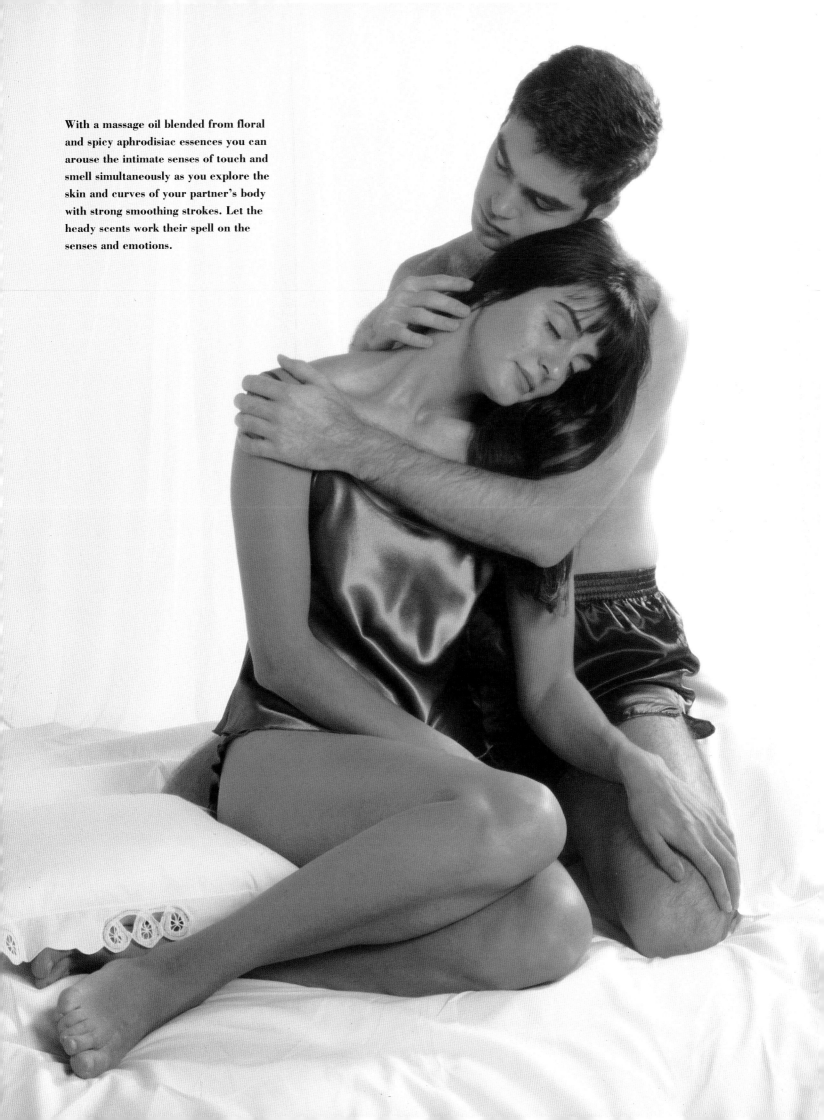

AMBIENT AROMAS

A lingering smell, whether pleasant or foul, is usually the first thing we notice when we enter a room, and it can strongly affect the way we feel. Fragrancing the home to cover unpleasant smells and delight the senses is an old tradition. For centuries the Chinese have suspended balls of jasmine flowers over the bed to clear the air and promote pleasant dreams, while posies of jasmine were handed to guests to refresh them on leaving banquets or dances. Lavender sachets placed in drawers and bowls of pot pourri to scent a room were particular favourites of the Victorians.

STUDIES AND OFFICES

Work-places are often stuffy and full of unpleasant smells, but if you work in an open-plan space fragrancing the whole area may not be a viable option. Inhaling a few drops of oil from a handkerchief is the most personal way of using a fragrance, or you can spray your immediate environment with a room spray, or add a couple of drops of oil to a cup of hot water on your desk.

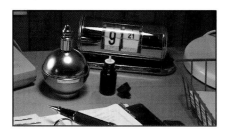

Useful oils for the work-place are basil, rosemary, bergamot, lemon and melissa. Bergamot and lemon are particularly antiseptic, and lemon has the added advantage of helping efficiency. Basil stimulates a tired brain and rosemary is a great aid to concentration. Rosemary is also helpful in relieving headaches. If you are feeling overwrought try clary sage or juniper, but watch the dosage as too much will cause sleepiness.

LIVING ROOMS

The methods for fragrancing a room are many and diverse. Those that involve evaporating the oils, such as fragrancers/diffusers, water bowls, light-bulb rings and room sprays, are best for preventing ill-health, balancing the emotions and disguising unpleasant smells such as cigarette smoke or cooking odours. All these methods disperse the fragrance through a large space extremely quickly and effectively. For more lingering and subtle scents, blend your own pot pourri or, alternatively, use pomanders.

Rose, geranium, orange and lavender are pleasing and uplifting scents for a room, used individually or blended together.

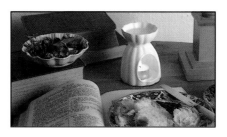

For an exotic, intimate atmosphere use sandalwood or patchouli, or to unwind in the evening try geranium, lavender, sandalwood or ylang-ylang.

Perfumes for parties

Clary sage or jasmine will create a heady, "feel-good" atmosphere for a party, or use orange, lemongrass or neroli for a lighter, fresher touch.

For a festive blend choose from the spicier oils such as frankincense, cedarwood, sandalwood, cinnamon and orange.

BEDROOMS

Whether to ensure a restful night's sleep or to turn your bedroom into a place of passion, fragrancing the bedroom just before retiring will create an appropriate atmosphere. Rose, neroli and lavender are delightful all-purpose oils for the bedroom. Use lavender to freshen a musty spare room to make it welcoming for guests.

INSECT REPELLANT

Use tea tree, eucalyptus, melissa, lemon grass or the closely related citronella in a diffuser to keep insects at bay.

DISINFECTING

Vaporized molecules of any essential oil will neutralize airborne bacteria, but some – such as tea tree, bergamot, lemon, pine and lavender – are particularly antiseptic. Use these in a fragrancer or room spray. Pine, lemon and tea tree can be used on a damp cloth to disinfect surfaces in the kitchen or bathroom. Clear the atmosphere of a sickroom with bergamot, eucalyptus and juniper.

POT POURRI

To make your own pot pourri assemble fully-dried flowers, petals, herbs, leaves and other plant materials. There are no hard and fast rules about quantities and proportions, but an allowance of two or three tablespoons ground spices, two tablespoons orris-root powder, two teaspoons dried lemon, orange or lime peel, and six drops of essential oil to every four cups of dried plant material makes a pleasant balanced mixture.

If your pot pourri loses a little of its aroma over a period of time, it can be revived. Simply stir in another two or three drops of essential oil. And if the mixture loses its colour sharpness just stir in a few dried flowers such as miniature rosebuds, santolina flowers or tansy clusters.

Cottage Garden Mix
1 cup dried lavender flowers
1 cup dried rose petals
1 cup dried pinks (*Dianthus*)
1 cup dried scented geranium leaves
1 tbsp (15g) ground cinnamon
2 tsp (10g) ground allspice
1 tsp (5g) dried grated lemon peel
2 tbsp (30g) orris-root powder
3 drops rose oil
3 drops geranium oil
Mix ingredients together in a covered container, and set aside for six weeks. Stir daily to distribute the fragrances.

Woodland Mix
1 cup lime seedpods, or "keys"
1 cup cedar bark shavings
1 cup sandalwood shavings
1 cup small cones
1 tbsp (15g) whole cloves
1 tbsp (15g) star anise
1 stick cinnamon, crushed
2 tbsp (30g) orris-root powder
4 drops sandalwood oil
2 drops cinnamon oil
Mix ingredients together in a covered container and set aside for six weeks. Stir daily.

Ingredients which can be used to make pot pourri. From the left: dried rosemary, lavender, and bay leaves, dried ground orris-root powder, dried rosemary leaves, a selection of essential oils, ground cinnamon, dried chilies and cinnamon sticks, whole cloves, a blend of dried flowers, limes and lemons. The dried peel of citrus fruit is finely grated or chopped for use in the spice mixture.

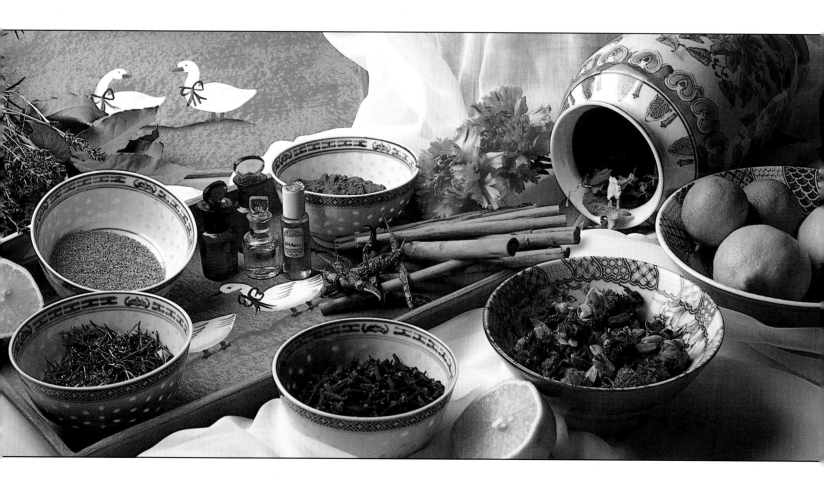

THE STRESS FACTOR

Pressure can be stimulating, challenging and motivating, but if it builds up we may be left feeling unable to cope. Our response is often to deny the pressure and ignore the physical signs of stress such as fatigue, self-doubt, sleeplessness and headaches. If the symptoms and causes of stress are left untreated they will affect your general health and well-being, and can even lead to serious illness, such as ulcers, heart attacks and clinical depression, so it's important to start tackling problems at an early stage, before they erupt. De-stressing requires a positive tactical plan for learning how to cope and retain a balanced outlook on life.

Aromatherapy is a marvellous antidote to many of the problems associated with stress as it draws on the calming, relaxing, uplifting and restorative powers of particular essential oils, providing a natural and powerful alternative to tranquillizers, anti-depressants and other drugs. They can work to relax the nervous system and give it enough stimulation to rebalance and control itself, leaving you refreshed and ready to cope.

ANXIETY

Whether it's a temporary bout of nerves, caused by something like an impending examination or interview, or an ongoing response to a persistent problem, anxiety can be a debilitating response to stress. It prevents you from dealing effectively with a problem and makes you feel tense. Essential oils, when inhaled, stimulate the lymbic portion of the brain which is responsible for all our feelings of well-being and discontent. They can balance the senses before deep depression sets into a more serious state. Temporary anxiety can also trigger skin eruptions so watch your diet and boost levels of vitamins C and E and B-complex.

Anxiety can be alleviated with a combination of uplifting and calming oils.

Basil (uplifting) · Bergamot (uplifting) · Geranium (relaxing) Lavender (soothing) · Neroli (sedative) · Sandalwood (calming)

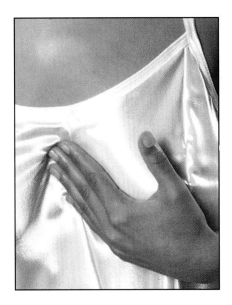

SOLAR PLEXUS STROKE

A marvellous way of unlocking tension by calming the main nerves that run through this area. Use your left hand (for calming) to stroke the solar plexus (located just below the breast bone) in anti-clockwise circles. Close your eyes as you do this and try to empty your mind. It can help soothe you even if you're clothed, but the effect is enhanced if you use a relaxing oil such as lavender or geranium. Try it while your bath is running, or when lying in bed before you go to sleep.

You can use the oils individually or mix them, using two relaxing oils to one uplifting oil. A good combination is basil, neroli and lavender. Stick to the same blend and proportions for bath and body, mixing five drops of each of the three oils in one tablespoon of base oil for the bath and two tablespoons for the body. All of the oils can be used individually in light-ring burners or fragrancers.

MILD SHOCK

This is a temporary form of stress, but the impact on the system can nonetheless be very strong, so a fast-acting remedy is needed.

Chamomile (calming) · Rosemary (stimulating) · Melissa (anti-depressant) · Neroli (relieves anxiety) · Peppermint (invigorating pain-reliever)

Use only two essential oils: both camphor and melissa work well individually with neroli, and peppermint has an affinity with melissa. Use a total of six drops in

1½ tablespoons of base oils, with smaller quantities of rosemary (for example, four drops of rosemary to six drops of melissa). For fast relief add four drops to a handkerchief and inhale.

HEADACHES

Often one of the first signs of stress and a regular affliction for many people. Cold compresses of lavender or geranium across the forehead provide pleasant relief. Add five drops of one oil to a small bowl of cool or warm water, soak a cloth in the water, wring out and lay it across the forehead. To help a headache caused by tension in the neck, try a sandalwood compress across the neck. Scalp massage is soothing, or try the shiatsu headache relief steps.

DEPRESSION

The blues can hit us all from time to time, as financial, emotional or work problems hang over like a dark cloud. In the long term, if problems are not resolved, depression lowers the immune system, leaving you prone to a spiral of worsening mental and physical health. Essential oils can work wonders in lifting the spirits to prevent this.

Uplifting Oils
Bergamot · Cypress · Lemongrass Rosemary · Sage

Soothing Oils
Chamomile · Geranium · Jasmine Lavender · Marjoram · Neroli Patchouli · Rose · Sandalwood Ylang-Ylang

Start off with three soothing oils, and then drop one of these in favour of an uplifting oil to give an element of stimulation, and eventually introduce two

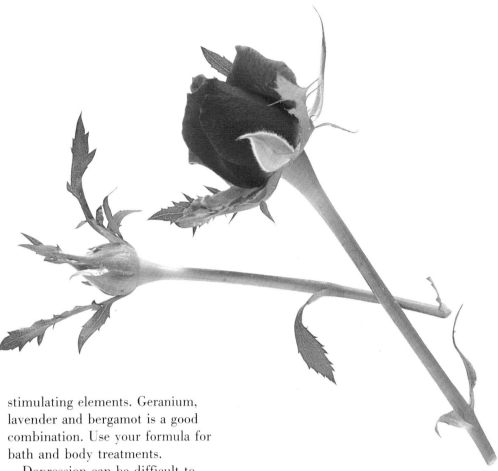

stimulating elements. Geranium, lavender and bergamot is a good combination. Use your formula for bath and body treatments.

Depression can be difficult to lift and if it persists you should consult a doctor or mental-health professional.

MENTAL FATIGUE

When you feel near to exhaustion or cannot concentrate on one thing at a time because problems seem to be crowding in on you, listen to your body's warning signals. Take time to unwind (try a bath with any of the soothing oils listed for depression), clear your head with a walk or deep-breathing exercises, and then revive yourself with oils such as eucalyptus and peppermint. Rosemary is helpful in concentrating the mind and stimulating the body so that you can continue to work if you feel you really can't afford to take a break.

INSOMNIA

Sleeplessness is a common response to stress, as your mind and body refuse to let go enough to give you the rest that you need. Learning to relax has to be built

into a daily pattern with a healthy diet, regular exercise, and a calming routine to wind down before bedtime. Try a milky drink or herbal tea last thing at night. Have a relaxing bath and massage, drawing on the sedative powers of up to three of the following oils:

Chamomile · Cedarwood Frankincense · Hyssop · Lavender Marjoram · Melissa · Neroli Orange · Patchouli · Rose · Sage Sandalwood · Ylang-Ylang

Breathing aromatic vapours in the bedroom helps to induce sleep:
Frankincense is warming and relaxing, and encourages tranquillity. Use in a fragrancer.
Lavender's relaxing quality can be harnessed by dabbing two drops on the edge of your pillow.
Marjoram has excellent soporific properties. Release in a light-bulb ring or fragrancer.
Neroli's wonderful floral fragrance is also sedative. Two drops on the pillow or in a fragrancer will help disperse unpleasant thoughts.

HEADACHE RELIEF

Headaches and migraines are common symptoms of stress. Follow these simple shiatsu steps to sweep away the tension, relieve pain and clear the head. The sequence is quick and easy to administer; it can be used anywhere and friends and colleagues will be grateful for the relief of their pain. You can perform some of the steps on yourself, though the healing touch of another's hands is more effective.

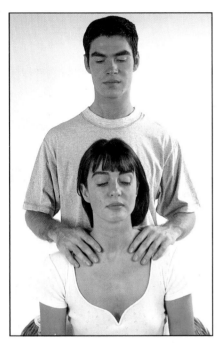

1 *Establish communication with your partner by placing both hands loosely on either side of the neck. Gently massage the shoulders; this helps to relax the breathing and creates a feeling of well-being.*

2 *Right: Tilt the head to the side and support with the palm of the hand so that the neck muscles can relax. Place the forearm across the shoulder and apply gentle downward pressure; hold for 5–10 seconds and then repeat with the other side. This movement is particularly good for opening the meridians running along the shoulders and neck.*

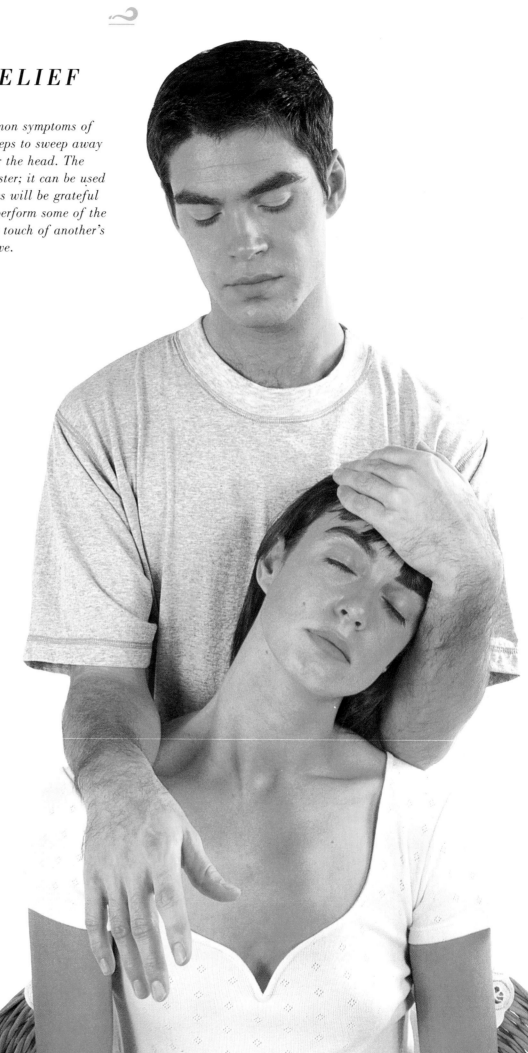

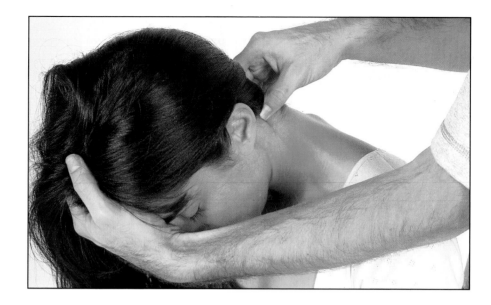

3 *Supporting the head with the left hand, work with thumb and forefinger applying gentle pressure from the base of the neck to the nape. Hold at the nape of the neck for five seconds and then release the built-up tension.*

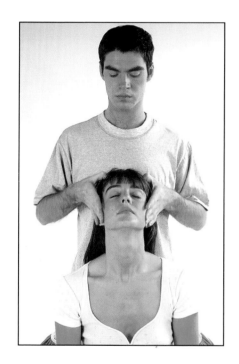

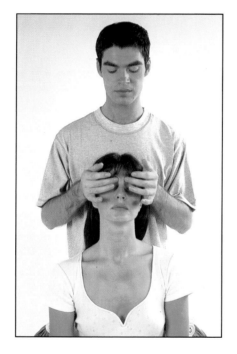

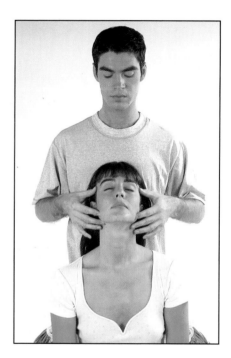

4 *Tilt the head back slightly, supporting it on your chest. Place your thumbs on the temples with the fingers loosely resting on either side of face. Gently rotate the thumbs in small forward movements.*

5 *Find the pressure points just above the inner corner of each eye. Apply gentle pressure with the middle fingers to help disperse the pain. Hold the pressure points for five seconds.*

6 *Position your thumbs on either side of the head just above the hairline – approximately two inches (5 cm) apart – with palms pressed flat along the sides of the face. Press the thumbs evenly back along the top of the head. This is a sensitive but invigorating movement to end the treatment.*

A shiatsu treatment is usually very effective for relieving stress and headaches but if your headache persists, consult a doctor. Avoid the treatment during pregnancy.

LEARNING TO RELAX

Relaxation is a prescription for health. Along with a well-balanced diet, an exercise programme, and a positive attitude towards recognizing and coping with stress, relaxation will help you balance the body and mind, even when you're worried and under pressure.

Exercise combats stress. The physically fitter you are, the better the body and mind can cope. Even burning off steam without losing self-control can be beneficial: a competitive racket sport, thumping the pillow, or going for a long walk can all release built-up tensions. Times of stress and emotional upset can make the body cry out for certain foods. Resist chocolate, cakes, ice cream or addictive stimulants like caffeine or nicotine. Feed the mind with a high intake of vitamin C from fresh fruit and vegetables, in particular citrus, berry and tropical fruits, and all of the B-complex vitamins.

WHOLE-BODY RELAXATION

Lie down straight with shoulders relaxed and even on the floor. Arms should be straight with elbows alongside the waist, palms turned upward. Relax your head and close the eyes. Breathe in deeply; allow your body to sink into the floor. Breathe out slowly; relax. Focus attention on your breathing; listen as you inhale and exhale and see how quiet the deep breathing can become.

Focus on breathing in and out, slowly and evenly.

Feet slightly apart and allowed to roll out naturally.

Let go of any tension in the knees.

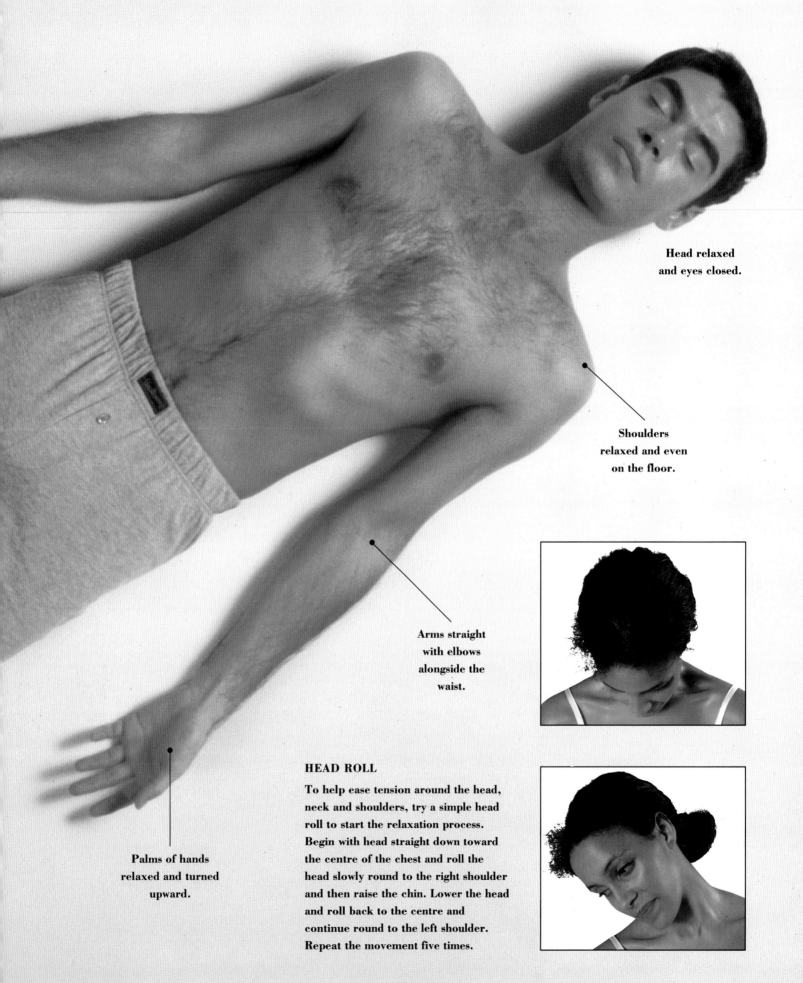

Head relaxed
and eyes closed.

Shoulders
relaxed and even
on the floor.

Arms straight
with elbows
alongside the
waist.

Palms of hands
relaxed and turned
upward.

HEAD ROLL

To help ease tension around the head,
neck and shoulders, try a simple head
roll to start the relaxation process.
Begin with head straight down toward
the centre of the chest and roll the
head slowly round to the right shoulder
and then raise the chin. Lower the head
and roll back to the centre and
continue round to the left shoulder.
Repeat the movement five times.

SHIATSU

The roots of shiatsu can be traced back over 5000 years to the ancient Chinese forms of medicine such as acupuncture and acupressure. However, it is a modern Japanese therapy, which fuses traditional Eastern practices with Western techniques of osteopathy. Literally translated the name means finger pressure – *Shi* (finger) and *Atsu* (pressure), although elbows, knees and feet are also used to press along the body's network of meridian lines and pressure points, releasing blocked channels of energy. It is an holistic method of alleviating pain and promoting health in the whole body.

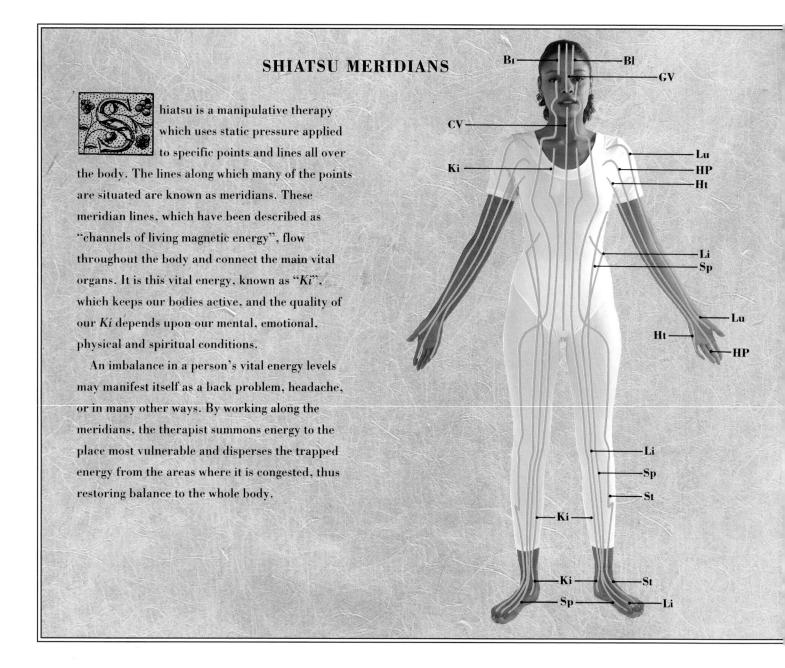

SHIATSU MERIDIANS

Shiatsu is a manipulative therapy which uses static pressure applied to specific points and lines all over the body. The lines along which many of the points are situated are known as meridians. These meridian lines, which have been described as "channels of living magnetic energy", flow throughout the body and connect the main vital organs. It is this vital energy, known as "*Ki*", which keeps our bodies active, and the quality of our *Ki* depends upon our mental, emotional, physical and spiritual conditions.

An imbalance in a person's vital energy levels may manifest itself as a back problem, headache, or in many other ways. By working along the meridians, the therapist summons energy to the place most vulnerable and disperses the trapped energy from the areas where it is congested, thus restoring balance to the whole body.

GIVING A SHIATSU SESSION

If your partner closes their eyes, this can make the session a special time to relax and switch off the world. There is no need to talk during a treatment as the communication of touch can say so much more. One of the fundamental principles of shiatsu is to have simultaneous touch from both hands. With a two-hand connection a circuit is created, bonding the giver and receiver. To keep this link, one hand is stationary – the support hand – and plays the role of listening and comforting your partner, while the other hand – the messenger hand – moves and does all the work. The amount of pressure from both hands will vary with the area of the body you are working on. The messenger and support hands change roles many times throughout a session. What you are trying to achieve is two points of contact merging and feeling like one to both therapist and partner.

Even as a beginner use your senses of looking, asking, listening and touching. Listen to your partner's needs and ask about symptoms before giving a treatment. Your motivation to help can be felt by your partner through the hands, transforming the simplest techniques into a caring bond. Before giving a shiatsu treatment, calm the mind, as any tension will transmit itself to your partner.

The Hara

The *Hara* is one of the most powerful energy centres of the body. In shiatsu terms it is known as the *Tanden*, and is located below the navel in the lower abdomen. It is the physical centre of the body and features prominently in all shiatsu treatments. The *Hara* incorporates the *Yin* (Earth) force flowing up the front of the body, and the *Yang* (Heaven) force flowing down the back merging into the lower abdomen. By focusing all movements from this centre, you can give harmonious and supportive treatments. Develop an open-posture principle in which your *Hara* is physically and energetically behind all your movements. This enables weight to be used instead of force. The simple rule is if you're not feeling comfortable and relaxed your partner will become aware of this.

Breathing is very important when stretching and applying pressure. Breathe in deeply and exhale as you move into a stretch, encouraging your partner to do the same.

Healing Energy

The aim of shiatsu is to balance the body's "*Ki*" energy levels. The rocking, kneading and stretching techniques are most effective in unblocking the congested areas. If your partner has a low energy

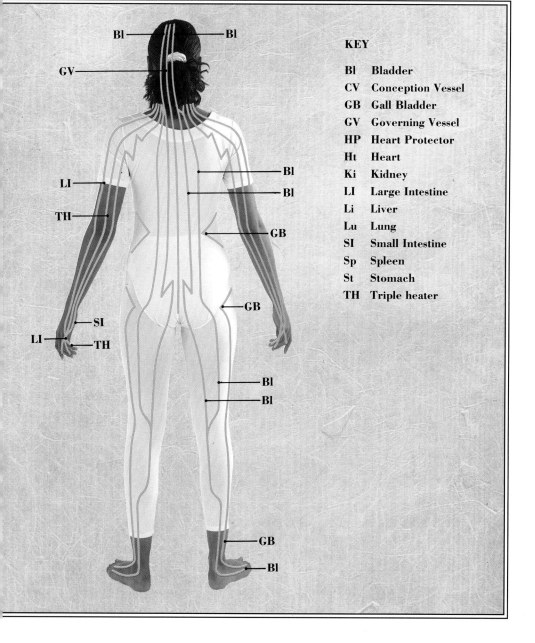

KEY

Bl	Bladder
CV	Conception Vessel
GB	Gall Bladder
GV	Governing Vessel
HP	Heart Protector
Ht	Heart
Ki	Kidney
LI	Large Intestine
Li	Liver
Lu	Lung
SI	Small Intestine
Sp	Spleen
St	Stomach
TH	Triple heater

level, and is generally fatigued, then slow, deep, static and perpendicular pressure will be more effective in strengthening the energy flow. Holding certain points from one to ten seconds is a general guideline but use your intuition as to how long you hold.

Practical Points

A shiatsu session normally lasts up to an hour. It is advisable to wear loose clothing so that your movements aren't hampered. The receiver is also clothed, but avoid bulky or constricting clothes that would impede contact with the body. Generally, the therapist works on the whole of the body and having discovered your problems may suggest simple practical exercises for home use to help the process of recovery. The effects of shiatsu may be felt immediately or later on in the same day, but if painful reactions are later experienced then your practitioner should be contacted. There are no two people with similar mental and physical complaints and the number of sessions will depend upon the individual's needs.

Shiatsu helps to keep open the communication between body, mind, emotion and spirit.

THE MAIN TECHNIQUES

PALMING

Palming is the simplest and most widely used technique in shiatsu. Palm pressure is gentle but firm, creating a supporting and soothing effect on any tense or vulnerable areas of the body.

Allow your hands to be relaxed so that your fingers can follow the contours of whatever part of the body you contact, then lean your body-weight through your palm, holding and waiting for the connection between your two palms. Lean back and without breaking contact, slide your hand along the body and lean forward again, creating stationary and perpendicular pressure.

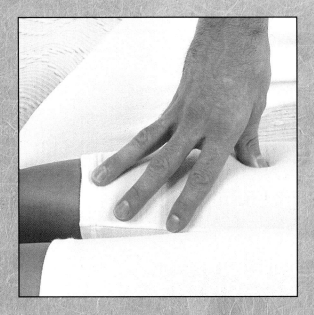

THUMBING

Thumb pressure is far more precise and penetrating than palming, and is used for working the points along the meridians. Place your thumbpads on the points. Use your extended fingers for support, so that the thumb remains straight. Lean your body forward so that most of the pressure is transferred through the thumbs. Make sure your nails are quite short to practise this technique or you may hurt your partner.

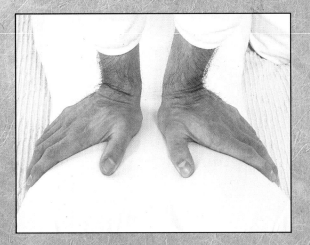

SIMPLE SHIATSU SESSION

The following sequences have been arranged so that each technique can flow smoothly into the next. Ideally the whole treatment should be experienced as a complete uninterrupted unit, not as a collection of separate movements. To achieve this, always maintain contact with your partner and make the transitions from one technique to the next with ease and fluency.

YANG

Position yourself at your partner's side. Take some time to centre yourself, clearing your mind so you can focus on your partner.

1 *Gently and firmly lay your hand on the small of your partner's back. This contact is an important time for both receiver and giver to attune to each other's energy. Use this time to assess the needs of your partner; feel the quality of the energy, physically, emotionally and spiritually. This can focus your intention in all the techniques to follow.*

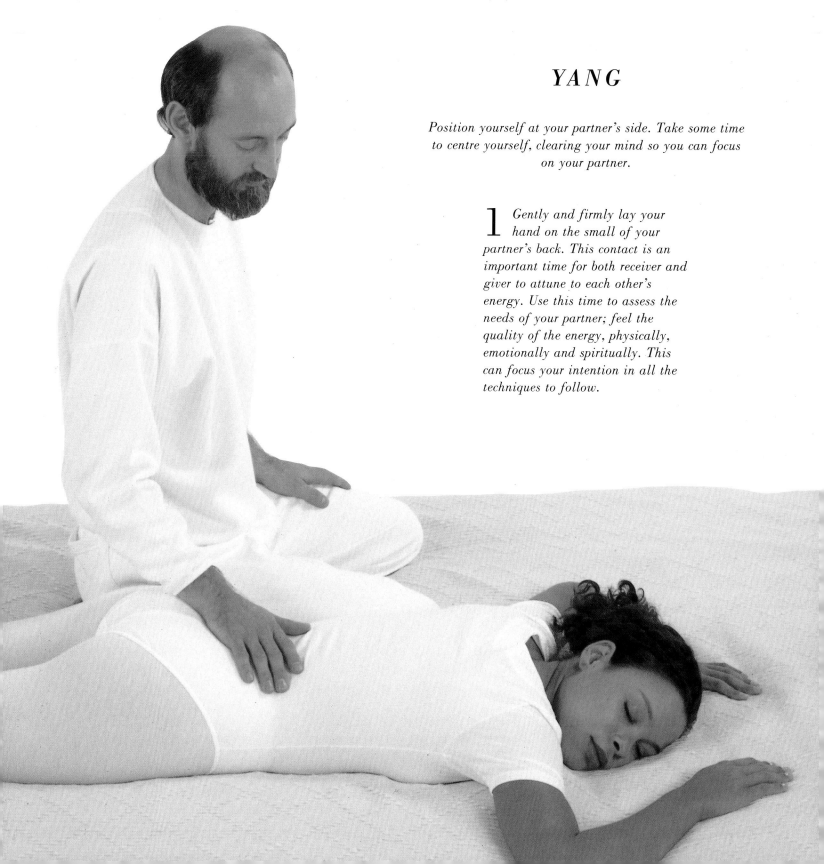

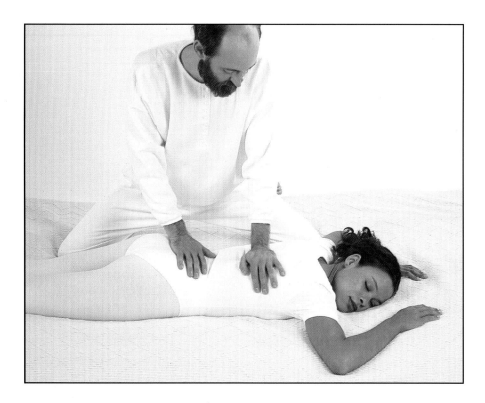

Left: This technique helps to disperse tension throughout, thus encouraging the energy to flow. It is useful to observe how your partner's body is moving. You will quickly be able to diagnose areas which may need more attention by simply observing which parts of the body are not moving as you rock.

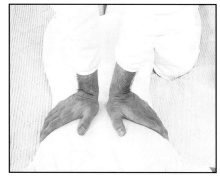

2 *Turn to face your partner and place the heel of the hands in the space between the shoulder blade and spine. With your knees apart begin to rock back and forth from your Hara (centre of the lower abdomen) and let the movement transfer through your hands so your partner's entire body moves in a*

wave-like motion. Continue to perform the rocking technique, working all the way down to the sacrum (lower back), moving the hands down the back in sequence.

Repeat two or three times and then repeat the same movements on the other side of the spine.

3 *Come up on to one knee, keeping an open posture. Placing your palms no higher than shoulder-blade level, on your receiver's "out" breath, bring your body-weight forward applying perpendicular pressure.*

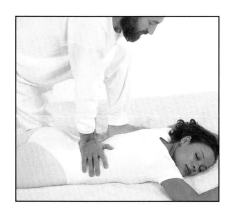

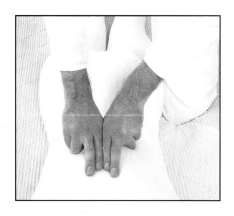

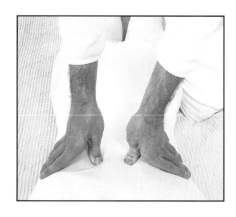

4 *Work down the back, moving a palm's width each time, and moving your body position to maintain perpendicular pressure. As you move below the ribs you may want to decrease the pressure slightly, as the internal organs are less protected here.*

5 *Having relaxed the back you can now locate the bladder meridian, which has a structural and energetic relationship with the nervous system. Measure two fingers' width from the centre of the spine and one hand's width down from the top of the shoulder.*

6 *Using the thumbs apply pressure at the points between the ribs. Thumb pressure is much more concentrated than palming. If you are unsure about how much pressure is appropriate, simply ask your partner how it feels.*

LEGS

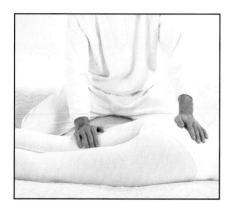

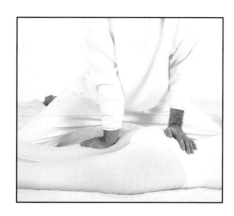

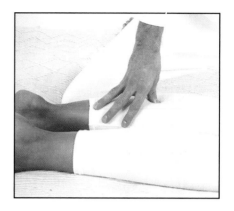

1 *Move your body down level to and facing your partner's legs. With your support hand on the lower back (sacrum), your messenger hand rocks and kneads simultaneously down the near-side thigh and calf several times.*

2 *Next palm down the leg, avoiding pressure on the backs of the knees.*

3 *Now thumb down the path of the bladder meridian. Depending on the length of the leg you may need to adjust your position. To avoid over-stretching, you can also move your support hand to just above the knee.*

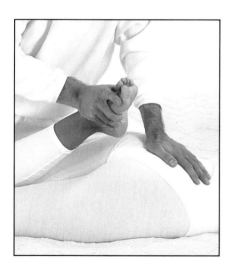

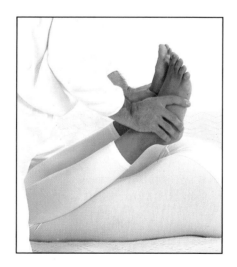

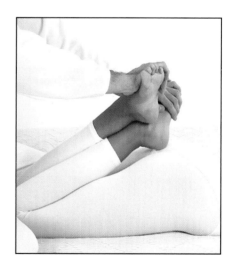

4 *With one hand on the sacrum, use the other hand to bring the foot gently back toward the buttocks, taking into consideration the leg's stretching capacity. Hold for a few seconds and then release.*

5 *Clasp both feet together and bend the legs, bringing the feet toward the buttocks. Hold this position for a few seconds and notice which foot goes closest to the buttocks to assess pelvic balance.*

6 *Cross this foot under the other foot and press them toward the buttocks on the "out" breath. Hold for several seconds then reverse the crossed legs and bend toward the buttocks once again.*

After these movements you will probably notice that the bending capacity of the legs has become more equal and the pelvis is more balanced.

Move round to the other side of the body and repeat the rocking, kneading, palming and thumbing on the other leg.

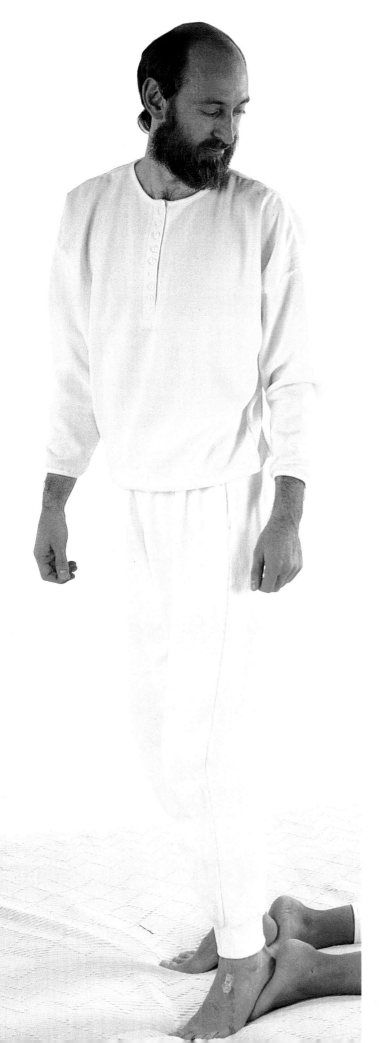

WORKING ON THE FEET

When "walking" on the feet make sure your position is well balanced as excess pressure or loss of balance may cause your partner pain.
Both the giving and receiving of pressure on the feet is very relaxing, and perfectly safe and easy to perform as long as you don't make any sudden or unexpected movements. Keep your body upright and relaxed as if you were going for a walk.
If there is too much of a gap between your partner's ankle and the floor, or the feet don't turn inward symmetrically, you may have to leave this technique out.

1 *Turn around so that your back is facing your partner and stand on both feet, shifting your weight from foot to foot. Control the movement from your hips.*

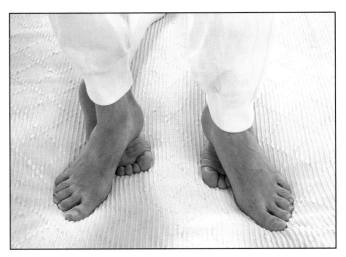

2 *Keep in one position and shift your weight back and forth from left to right several times and repeat on various areas of the feet.*

As with all the techniques, remember to observe your partner's facial expressions and breathing. These are obvious indications of how the receiver is feeling. Don't forget at any time that it's a human being you are working with, not just a body.
General pressure to the sole of the feet helps to stimulate the internal organs through the reflex areas and meridians. Walking on the feet is particularly good for grounding someone with too much mental activity.

YIN

Gently assist your partner to turn over into the supine position (on their back). Lying in this position we can be psychologically, emotionally and physically open, but we can also feel quite vulnerable. It is important to bear this in mind as you work to establish reassurance and trust.

Position yourself at your partner's side. Place one hand on your partner's waist, and the other hand on the abdomen with the heel of the hand just below the navel. Take a moment to listen with your hand to the rhythm of your partner's body. Feel the rise and fall of your partner's breath. Share the breath. This establishes a level of trust so

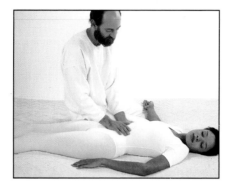

that you will be sensitive to any vulnerabilities or pains that might become manifest.

Gently palm around the abdomen in a clockwise direction. If you can coordinate your movements with your partner's "out" breath you should find that your partner gradually allows you to apply more pressure.

LEGS

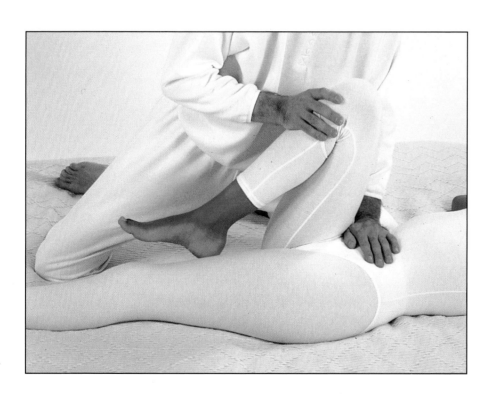

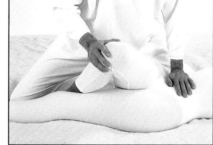

1 *Change your position to face across your partner, placing your uppermost hand on the Hara (lower abdomen). Place your other hand on the inside of the knee allowing your fingers to curl under*

the joint. Leaning back, simply allow your body weight to lift the leg. There should be very little effort involved in this. As the leg comes up, slide your hand from the inside of the knee to the upper shin.

2,3 *Rotate the leg out from the body, focusing on the hip joint. Start with small circular movements and, releasing the leg as much as possible, gradually increase the rotation to the fullest range.*

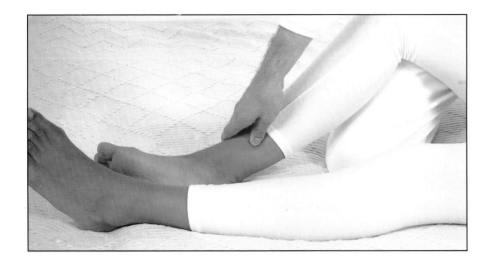

4 *Place the leg so that it rests comfortably with the toes at the level of the opposite ankle, with the spleen meridian uppermost. You may prop it up either with* your leg underneath or a cushion. Palm up the inside of the calf along the Yin *meridians to the knee. Thumb up the calf from the ankle to the knee.*

5 *Use your forearm to continue the pressure up the thigh. Rotate the leg once again then move down to your partner's feet.*

═══ **CAUTION** ═══

Do not give shiatsu on the spleen meridian during pregnancy if miscarriage is likely. Do not work below the knees in any pregnancy.

6 *Cup underneath the ankle in one hand. Place the other hand on top of the ankle. Bring your* Hara *into contact with the sole of the foot. Grasp it firmly and rotate your body from the hips. As you move your partner's body will move with yours.*

Repeat all the techniques on the opposite leg and complete this section of the sequence with your hand back on your receiver's Hara.

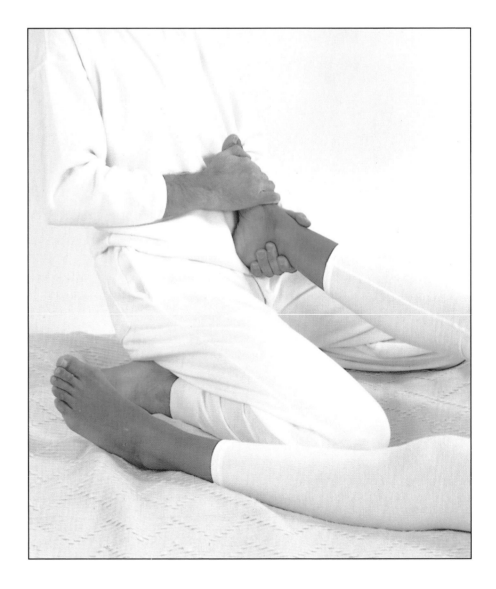

SHOULDERS, ARMS AND HANDS

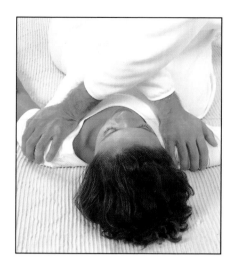

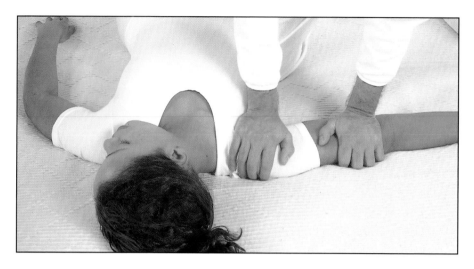

1 *Kneeling up, bring your free hand to your partner's furthest shoulder. Place your other hand on the near shoulder. Your arms should now be crossed. With your receiver's "out" breath, lean forward on your hands, opening up the shoulder and chest area.*

2 *Maintain the support of the shoulder nearest you. With the other hand, as in the treatment of the legs, begin by gently rocking and kneading the arms from the shoulder to the hand. Position the arm at right angles to the body*

with the palms facing up. Then palm down the arm, avoiding pressure on the elbow joint. Follow by thumbing down the middle of the arm to the palm along the heart protector meridian.

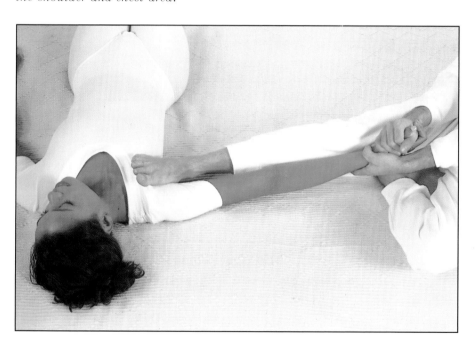

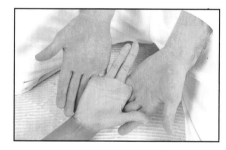

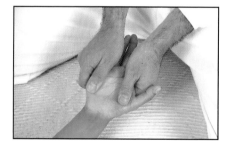

3 *Grasp the wrist and move your body so that your outstretched leg is parallel to the arm, your foot resting comfortably against the*

upper torso. Gently lean back stretching the arm, giving counterpressure with your foot.

4,5 *Link your little fingers inside your partner's index and little finger to stretch open the palm. Your thumbs are then naturally placed to work into the palm with circular movements.*

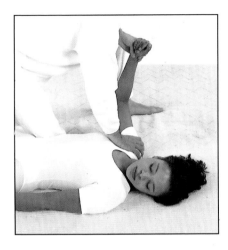

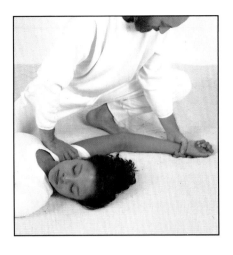

6 *Place the support hand on the shoulder, tucking your thumb into the armpit. Hold the wrist, lift and loosen the shoulder joint.*

7 *Step forward with your outside leg, stretching your partner's arm to the floor above the head.*

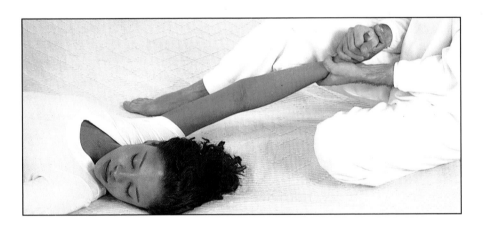

8 *Move your body so that by gently leaning back your* partner's arm is stretched, using a two-handed grip to the wrist.

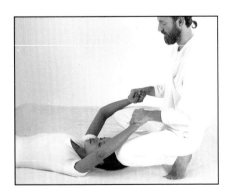

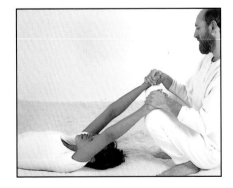

9 *Pick up your partner's other hand and rest the forearms on your knees.*

10 *Lean back, allowing your knees to slide up the forearms to the wrists. On the "out" breath, this makes a powerful stretch for the shoulders and chest.*

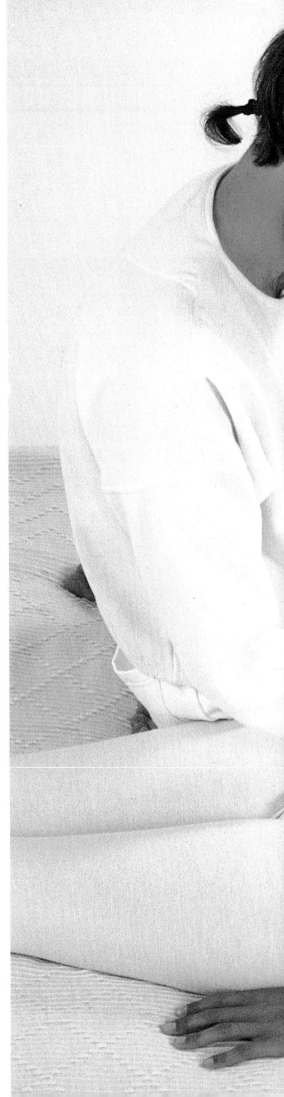

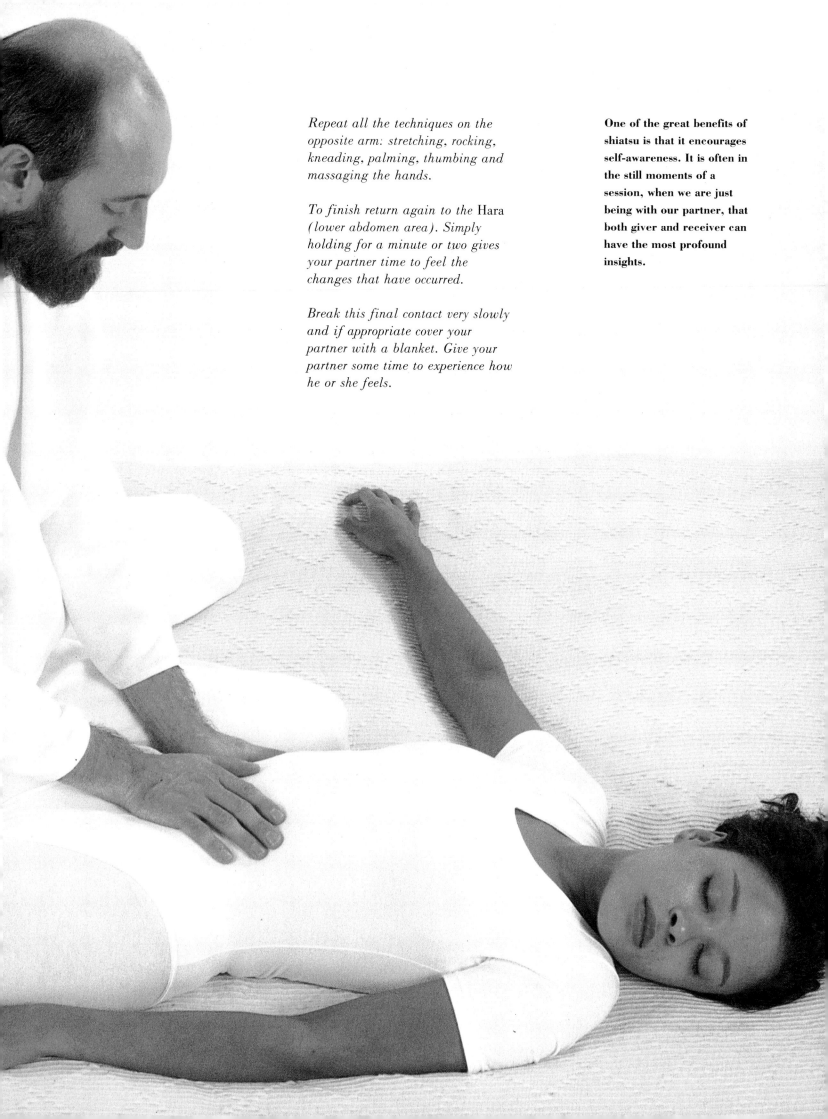

Repeat all the techniques on the opposite arm: stretching, rocking, kneading, palming, thumbing and massaging the hands.

To finish return again to the Hara (lower abdomen area). Simply holding for a minute or two gives your partner time to feel the changes that have occurred.

Break this final contact very slowly and if appropriate cover your partner with a blanket. Give your partner some time to experience how he or she feels.

One of the great benefits of shiatsu is that it encourages self-awareness. It is often in the still moments of a session, when we are just being with our partner, that both giver and receiver can have the most profound insights.